The Wounded Healer

The Wounded Healer

Addiction-Sensitive Approach to the Sexually Exploitative Professional

Richard Irons, M.D.
Jennifer P. Schneider, M.D.

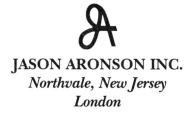

JASON ARONSON INC.
Northvale, New Jersey
London

This book was set in 11 pt. New Baskerville.

Library of Congress Cataloging-in-Publication Data

Irons, Richard, M.D.
    The wounded healer : addiction-sensitive approach to the sexually
exploitative professional / by Richard Irons and Jennifer Schneider.
        p. cm.
    Includes bibliographical references.
    ISBN 1-56821-763-3
    1. Sex between psychotherapist and patient. 2. Psychotherapists—
Mental health. 3. Psychotherapists—Sexual behavior.
4. Psychotherapists—Counseling of. 5. Psychiatrists—Professional
ethics. 6. Sex addiction—Treatment. 7. Sexually abused patients.
I. Schneider, Jennifer P.   II. Title.
    [DNLM: 1. Behavior, Addictive—therapy. 2. Sex Offenses—
psychology. 3. Psychotherapy—methods. 4. Professional–Patient
Relations. 5. Professional Impairment—psychology. WM 176 I71w
1999]
RC489.S47I76   1998
616.89'14—DC21
DNLM/DLC
for Library of Congress   98-21444

Printed in the United States of America on acid-free paper. For information and catalog write to Jason Aronson Inc., 230 Livingston Street, Northvale, New Jersey 07647-1726. Or visit our website: http://www.aronson.com

To the memory of my father, Raphael Patai, 1910–1996—cultural anthropologist, teacher, and author. By his lifelong example, he taught me both the value and the pleasure of scholarship.

—Jennifer Schneider

To the memory of my father, Earl Jilson Irons Jr., 1927–1992, purple heart survivor of the Normandy invasion and carpenter, and his father, Earl Jilson Irons 1900–1970, veteran and mason; they taught me to believe that with effort and perseverance, determination and belief in what is true, great things may be accomplished.

—Richard Irons

Contents

PART III: HEALING THE WOUNDED

Introduction

Relationships between helping professionals (such as doctors, counselors, lawyers, ministers, or teachers) and those they serve have always been seen as having special significance and meaning. They have been circumscribed and set apart by ritual and professional ethics as protected and sacred, and the basis of service within the profession. The covenant between the professional and the individual served is inherent, and follows from the Latin dictum *primum non nocere* (first, do no harm).

Yet professionals are as human as those they serve. Sexual relationships and other improprieties occur between such persons in power and those they serve. Though such scenarios may be prime material for high drama in books, movies, and exposés, virtually all such "romances" are destructive not only for the protagonists but also for their families. Relationships between persons of unequal power are a significant cause of psychological distress, shattered marriages and careers, legal problems, and even imprisonment.

The literature in the fields of psychology and psychiatry contains an increasing number of first-person accounts of victims, recommendations for treatment of the victims, and theories about why persons in power take sexual advantage of others. Yet there is ongoing disagreement about what constitutes sexual abuse of a professional relationship and whether the person with lesser power can actually give informed consent to the relationship. In particular, there is a paucity of information to help clinicians understand and manage a professional who has had sexual contact with a patient or client. Unlike previous books and articles dealing with the trauma experienced by victims of sexual exploitation, the present volume seeks to address the causes of sexual exploitation and their implications for assessment and treatment of the victimizer. Helping clinicians work with exploitative professionals is the goal of this book.

The authors' own professional journeys led them independently to work with themes of male exploitation of power in such relationships, and to combine their experience in ongoing collaboration over the past seven years. They are both board-certified internal medicine specialists with a subspecialty and certification in addiction medicine.

Richard Irons currently serves as the associate program director of the Addiction Recovery Program at the Menninger Clinic in Topeka, Kansas. He supervises a program for assessing and treating professionals who present with allegations of professional sexual impropriety or offense.

After working with state licensure boards and professional associations in supervising assessment and treatment of chemically dependent health care professionals for seven years, Irons was recruited by Golden Valley Hospital, a psychiatric hospital in Minneapolis, to develop a dedicated program to assess helping professionals who were facing allegations of professional sexual misconduct. Golden Valley had become nationally known for its work in the treatment of addictive sexual disorders. It often received inquiries from regulatory agencies and other concerned parties requesting evaluation of questionable behavior on the part of a professional who denied any wrongdoing. The author developed a multidisciplinary assessment program that subsequently moved to

Abbott Northwestern Hospital and continues to function, providing a variety of assessment services for professionals.

Over the past ten years, Irons has served as an assessment provider to more than thirty-six state licensure boards and five provincial colleges in Canada. He has served as a consultant for numerous professional regulatory agencies and associations in developing strategies and policies for addressing professional sexual misconduct, and in preparing guidelines for professional reentry when such action is deemed safe and appropriate. During this time, he has been directly involved in the assessment of over 350 helping professionals facing allegations of professional sexual impropriety or misconduct. At the Menninger Clinic, he is directly involved in the provision of treatment, therapy, and continuing care to professionals with a variety of personal and professional problems.

In his clinical experience with professionals facing allegations of professional sexual misconduct, Irons found that many had cognitive distortions and self-defeating behavior with an admixture of compulsive and impulsive features that closely paralleled the presentation of substance dependence. In fact, a significant minority, about 37 percent, met the diagnostic criteria for substance abuse or dependence. More than half of the professionals Schneider and Irons (1996) studied in a review of 137 consecutive professionals presenting with allegations of professional sexual misconduct had sexual disorders with defined addictive features.

Eventually, Irons proposed an archetypal typology of male professionals who engaged in professional misconduct or offense. The typology was based on the experiential determination that different patterns of exploitation required different treatment and therapy, and often differed substantially in their prognosis for professional rehabilitation and return to duty. When an addictive disorder was present, primary and continuing addiction treatment and care was indicated. When significant characterological pathology or dysfunction was present, then insight-oriented psychotherapy was usually necessary and the path to personal healing and at times professional rehabilitation was often prolonged. Cognitive-behavioral treatment was needed in other situations where the patterns of exploitation were more regressed and ingrained, especially when paraphilias were present. Major mental disorders on Axis I of the *Diagnostic and Statistical Manual of Mental Disorders (DSM-IV* 1994) required appropriate treatment and ongoing care, including pharmacotherapy.

Appropriate, effective treatment of the sexually exploitative professional requires the initial creation of a comprehensive database, and a multidisciplinary assessment is an efficient and rapid means to accomplish this task. Treatment of the professional and the victim(s) of such sexual misconduct requires time and much effort. Healing does eventually come to most of those touched by this painful and unfortunate complication that stems from relationships based on unequal power and the need for privacy and trust. Not all professionals who have engaged in such misconduct could or should return to professional practice. Strict criteria, such as those proposed by the authors, have been used as guidelines by licensure boards and regulatory agencies to protect the public when such professionals are permitted to return to professional duties. Finally, we all need to recognize that the majority of the victims of professional sexual misconduct and their families receive far less, if any, treatment and therapy compared to the professionals. This injustice needs to be addressed at every turn.

Jennifer Schneider is the medical director of Kachina Center for Addiction Recovery, an outpatient treatment center in Tucson, Arizona, and has an office-based practice in internal medicine and addiction medicine. A holder of a Ph.D. in genetics, her academic orientation led her to begin research in addictive sexual disorders in the late 1980s particularly in the areas of recovery for family members and for couples dealing with sexual addiction problems.

Like so many other professionals in the addiction field, Schneider's interest was sparked by a personal experience, in her case having learned in 1983 of the presence of an addictive sexual problem in a family member. At that time a practicing internist, she began to study the field of chemical dependency in order to understand how a behavior can be addictive. Very little was written then about behavior addictions, but the parallels with chemical dependency, both in the addict and in family members, were very clear to her. Hundreds of self-identified sex addicts and their spouses or partners who were members of self-help programs based on the Alcoholics Anonymous and Al-Anon models became participants in her research. She also began receiving referrals from psychiatrists and therapists in the community for assessment of addictive sexual disorders.

Chemical dependency clinicians have long been aware that even when a professional's personal life is falling apart because of an addiction, he or she will try as long as possible to keep the addiction out of the workplace. Thus, a physician who comes to work intoxicated is usually already in an advanced stage of alcoholism. Similarly, in reviewing the history of a professional's sexually addictive behavior, it was clear to Schneider that involvement with patients or clients was usually preceded by other compulsive sexual behaviors outside the workplace. In other words, sexual exploitation of multiple patients or clients by a professional is usually a sign of an advanced stage of an addictive sexual disorder. The traditional response to sexual impropriety—temporary suspension of a professional license; some other punishment, such as a fine; or transfer to another position (the historical approach to clergy sexual misconduct)—is unlikely to stop the behavior. Only recognition of the real nature of the problem, followed by appropriate treatment, makes it possible in some cases for the professional to safely return to practice. When an addictive disorder has been diagnosed, appropriate treatment is not individual psychotherapy but rather addiction treatment and the recognition that addiction is a chronic and potentially relapsing condition that requires ongoing attention to recovery.

After finding themselves presenting at the same professional conferences on several occasions, the two authors decided to collaborate. The current work is the distillation of what they have learned. It is presented to provide the psychotherapy clinician with a framework for approaching a colleague or client who admits to or is accused of a sexual impropriety. Even clinicians trained in both addiction and psychiatry cannot be expected to duplicate the assessment program described in this book, but the reader will glean enough to recognize that sexually exploitative behavior has several possible causes, addiction being prominent among them, and will be able to make appropriate referrals for assessment and treatment.

Section I provides the reader with a framework to facilitate understanding appropriate boundaries and recognizing the nature and scope of sexual exploitation. Chapter 1 reviews the scope of the problem of sexual exploitation by health professionals and clergy, defines professional sexual misconduct and sexual offense, and describes the assessment program created by Irons and the causes of sexual exploitation found among the first 150 professionals assessed.

Because understanding the concept of boundaries is critical to recognizing when a professional has been exploitative, Chapter 2 discusses boundaries, how they develop, and how boundary problems can lead to sexual exploitation. The emphasis is on male development, since the vast majority of sexually exploitative professionals are male.

To facilitate understanding of the relationship between sexual disorders and addictive disease, Chapter 3 begins with an overview of sexual disorders as catalogued in the fourth edition of the *DSM-IV* (1994); this will undoubtedly be familiar to many readers. However, most readers will welcome the discussion on diagnosis of addiction in general and of an addictive behavioral disorder in particular. We also provide a list of types of addictive sexual behaviors and how they relate to the *DSM-IV*. A differential diagnosis of excessive sexual behaviors is also presented to provide a framework for understanding specific cases of sexual impropriety.

It is clearly improper for a person in power to coerce another person into sexual activity. But what about apparently consensual sex between a doctor and patient, or therapist and client? What about consensual sex with a former patient or client? Clinicians as well as laymen often have difficulty deciding what is ethical and what is not, what is consensual and what is not. This is the subject of Chapters 4 and 5, which explain the nature of sexual exploitation, the role of transference and countertransference in therapeutic relationships, who is particularly vulnerable to sexual exploitation, and the likely effect on the victim. This is the only discussion of victims, as the focus of the book is primarily on the perpetrator; the treatment of victims is being increasingly addressed in the professional psychological literature.

Separating sexually exploitative men into an archetypal framework has been helpful in making treatment recommendations as well as in determining the risk of recurrence. Section II provides descriptions of each of the six archetypes created by Irons. After an introduction in Chapter 6, they are detailed in Chapters 7 through 12, which describe specific cases and how they were treated.

Once the reader understands the nature and variations of sexual exploitation, Section III attempts to delineate an approach to recovery, both for the professional himself and for his spouse. When sexual exploitation comes to light, attention is focused on the exploitative professional and on the victim, but another victim is usually forgotten—the professional's spouse or significant other. Recovering addicts are less likely to relapse, and their families are more likely to stay intact, when the spouse's concerns are recognized and the spouse participates in the treatment plan. Similarly, incarcerated sex offenders and other prison inmates are less likely to reoffend when contact is maintained with their families. Chapter 13 describes the effects of sexual exploitation on the offender's wife. We hope that clinicians will recognize the need to attend to this secondary victim.

Finally, Chapter 14 reviews some archetypal themes, summarizes our observations on the stages through which exploitative professionals pass on the path to wholeness, and discusses the challenges entailed in fulfilling the role of a helping professional.

This book is the collaboration of two authors. Although both authors had input into each chapter, Dr. Schneider was primarily responsible for Section I and Chapter 13, while Dr. Irons penned most of Section II and Chapter 14. The stylistic differences of the two authors will be evident to the reader. The authors believe that the different content of their writing is appropriately reflected in the different tones they chose to use. For this reason, they decided against attempting to force a uniform style to the book, and they beg the reader's indulgence in adapting to the differences in tone.

The cases described in this book are based on real people. However, details have been changed to preserve their anonymity and some case reports are composites of more than one individual. Except for Dr. Margaret Bean-Bayog, a public figure, all other names are fictitious.

Part I

Toward an Understanding of Sexual Exploitation

1

Sexual Exploitation: Definition and Assessment

In every house where I come I will enter only for the good of my patients, keeping myself far from all intentional ill-doing and all seduction, and especially free from the pleasure of love with women or with men.

Excerpt from the *Hippocratic Oath*

Since the time of Hippocrates it has been recognized that the unique nature of the physician–patient relationship is threatened and distorted by intimate emotional or sexual contact within this relationship. The Hippocratic Oath specifically warns against sexual involvement with patients, yet it commonly occurs. Why does this happen? Why do some professionals suddenly or repeatedly abuse their power and position? Once caught and made to face the consequences of their behavior, can these professionals ever safely return to practice? Or is punishment, civil litigation, or termination of a career society's only recourse?

We begin with a review of survey findings on the prevalence of sexual involvement in asymmetric relationships, and then turn to a more intensive assessment to learn about the exploiters' motivations, psychopathology, and prognosis. This chapter presents the results of an intensive multidisciplinary assessment of more than 200 clergy, lawyers, and licensed health professionals who were accused of sexual misconduct or sexual offense. This assessment process has yielded some surprising answers to the questions posed above.

The inherent disparity in position, education, and power between a professional and a patient is an integral part of the healing that occurs in the therapeutic relationship. Each patient or client attempts to muster the courage and faith to trust the professional and implement the instructions and counsel given. The trust, however, is not always deserved.

Since the beginning of recorded history there have been standards of conduct and ethical codes established for those given the privilege to serve others. Healers are human, however, and therefore subject to the same maladies and shortcomings as their patients. Though held to a higher moral and ethical standard, they sometimes fail to attain perfection in the discharge of duties. Abuse of power and position for control and personal gain within the professional–client relationship has been recognized since ancient times, as documented by warnings, admonitions, and codes of conduct that can be found in virtually all major cultures and professional traditions.

Sexual exploitation by a person in power is an ancient theme in art and literature, a theme to which high school students are often first exposed in the novel The Scarlet Letter, by Nathaniel Hawthorne, a story of a young woman who takes all the blame for her sexual relationship with a minister. Currently, interest in this theme is at all-time high. In the book and film The Prince of Tides, a psychiatrist has an affair with the brother of her patient, but the story makes it clear that she is also providing him with therapy. The film Final Analysis describes the unfortunate consequences for a male psychiatrist who gets involved with the sister of a patient, but does not raise the issue of the impropriety of his involvement.

Once thought to be rare, childhood sexual abuse, the most frequent prototype of sexual exploitation by a person in power, is now considered to be so common that it is claimed that one in four children is a victim of incest or molestation. The destructive impact of such childhood experiences is often expressed in adulthood as sexual dysfunction, difficulty trusting others, avoidance of intimacy, and addiction to drugs or sexual behaviors. For example, approximately 80 percent of female alcoholics are believed to have been sexually abused during their childhood.

Sexual exploitation of adults by other adults in greater power is often analogous to incest, as we will demonstrate later. The helping professions uniformly condemn sexual relations between professionals and clients. The Council on Ethical and Judicial Affairs of the American Medical Association concluded in 1991 that "sexual contact or a romantic relationship with a patient concurrent with the physician–patient relationship is unethical. Sexual or romantic relationships with former patients are also unethical if the physician uses or exploits trust, knowledge, emotions, or influence derived from the previous professional relationship" (p. 2741).

The Ethics Committee of the American Psychiatric Association (1986) noted that "the necessary intensity of the therapeutic relationship may tend to activate sexual and other needs and fantasies on the part of both patient and therapist," but concludes, "Sexual activity with a patient is unethical" (p. 5).

Professional religious associations similarly condemn sexual relations between clergyperson and parishioner. The code of the American Association of Pastoral Counselors (Fortune 1989) states, "Pastoral counselors do not engage in sexual misconduct with their clients" (p. 84). The nature of the sexual misconduct is not specified. The Code of Professional Ethics of the Unitarian-Universalist Ministers Association (1993) prohibits "sexual activity with . . . a counselee, with the spouse or partner of a person in the congregation, with interns, or any other such exploitative relationship" (p. 7).

In Minnesota it is a felony for a counselor to engage in sexual activity with a client. This is also true in several other states, including Wisconsin and North Dakota.

PREVALENCE OF SEXUAL IMPROPRIETY

Despite condemnation by ethical codes of all the helping professions, sexual misconduct and offense are among the most common and most egregious violations of power and position. Surveys show that such abuse is much more common than has been recognized. For example, in an anonymous survey of over 1,300 psychiatrists (Gartrell et al. 1986), 6.4 percent acknowledged having had sexual contact with their own patients; one-third of this group had been involved with more than one patient. Sexual contact was defined as "physical contact that arouses or satisfies sexual desire in the patient, physician, or both" (p. 139). Gartrell and colleagues found that repeat offenders were particularly likely to believe in the therapeutic value of sexual relations with patients, and to believe that sexual relations would provide a corrective emotional experience, or would change a patient's sexual orientation. They seemed particularly unable to recognize the harmfulness of their behavior, even though this is generally accepted.

In a follow-up anonymous survey of almost 1,900 family practitioners, obstetrician-gynecologists, internists, and surgeons (Gartrell et al. 1992), 9 percent acknowledged sexual contact with at least one patient. This group consisted of 10 percent of all the male physicians and 4 percent of the females. Other surveys of psychotherapists and social workers have yielded similar results. The prevalence of sexual exploitation by priests and ministers is harder to evaluate, but the increasing publicity and mounting legal costs for the Catholic Church and other churches attests to the growing problem. It appears that approximately 6 to 9 percent of helping professionals have violated the codes of ethics of their profession by having sexual contact with a patient or client at some point in their careers. In doing so they have knowingly damaged their clients and have risked losing their license, career, reputation, families, and, in some cases, their freedom.

DEFINITION OF TERMS

In the reports of anonymous surveys, respondents admitted to various types of sexual impropriety. We have developed definitions for the types of behaviors described in this book:

Professional sexual misconduct is defined as the overt or covert expression of erotic or romantic thoughts, feelings, or gestures by the professional toward the patient or client, that are sexual or may reasonably be construed by the patient as sexual.

Sexual offense is defined as a nontherapeutic, nondiagnostic attempt by the professional to touch, or have any actual contact with, any of the anatomic areas of the patient's body commonly considered reproductive or sexual.

The array of conduct we are discussing includes sexual innuendo and derogatory comments, verbal and physical improprieties such as nontherapeutic hugs, erotically charged encounters with a patient in or out of the office, romantic enmeshment with a patient, sexual involvement with a family member of a patient, medical voyeurism or exhibitionism or nontherapeutic touch, unnecessary or prolonged genital examination, a surgeon offering "sexually enhancing" procedures, a therapist offering sexual relations with a patient in order to solve the patient's sexual or relationship problems, and sexual molestation of a patient who is physically, mentally, or emotionally unable to offer resistance or is unconscious or under the influence of mood-altering substances. This is a highly charged emotional, moral, and legal terrain filled with many ambiguities and gray zones.

As we are defining these terms, *sexual misconduct* and *sexual offense* refer only to behaviors between the professional and the client. When similar behavior—sexual innuendoes, unwanted advances, physical improprieties—occur between the professional and a member of the office or hospital staff, we recognize that they are still exploitative, but we refer to those incidents as sexual harassment rather than as sexual misconduct or offense. These behaviors often overlap, however; many professionals who sexually exploit their clients are also likely to sexually exploit their staff.

THE PROFESSIONAL ASSESSMENT PROGRAM

Data obtained from anonymous statistical surveys do not yield insights into the reasons that professionals take these risks. Only in-depth psychological evaluations of individuals can give such answers, as well as provide prognostic information on the risk of repeat offending. Over the past several years, Irons has carried out such evaluations of over 200 physicians, psychologists, clergy, and other helping professionals. We will describe this program in order to demonstrate the thoroughness that we believe the evaluation of difficult cases requires and to show what we learned from the patients who went through the program. Other similar programs are now available in other parts of the United States.

The Professional Assessment Program, originally located in Minneapolis, Minnesota, is a short-term inpatient process that provides multidisciplinary assessment for possible impairment associated with allegations of sexual misconduct or sexual offense. As an intensive, multidisciplinary program, it was developed in response to the needs expressed by licensure boards, regulatory agencies, and professional societies to have an objective forum in which allegations of sexual impropriety could be explored and considered independent of treatment, administrative due process, civil suits, and criminal legal process. It is an alternative or supplementary means by which an accused professional may come to consider possible the personal vulnerabilities and errors in judgment that may have contributed to the complaints or allegations that have been brought forward. Most patients are referred by their state professional regulatory board.

The five-day inpatient assessment is useful for cases where the allegations are disputed or imprecise, or where the case is complex and the diagnosis unclear. In straightforward cases where the professional acknowledges the alleged sexual impropriety, a briefer outpatient evaluation by a psychologist or psychiatrist may suffice.

The goals of the assessment program are:

- to reconstruct the events leading to assessment;
- review past corrective actions, previous evaluations, and treatment;
- assist the patient in making appropriate self-diagnoses;

- break through defenses that prevent the patient from recognizing the nature of his problems and the need for change;
- establish a causal hypothesis that helps to explain past actions, and provide diagnostic conclusions and recommendations for the future; and
- encourage the patient to formulate and implement a plan following discharge.

The crucial objective in assessment is to establish a causal hypothesis that helps explain the reasons for the complaints, and the behavior of the professional patient.

Prior to admission, we request from concerned parties and referral sources all available information on the professional including the allegations and complaints that are known. We are unwilling to proceed with an assessment unless we have a reliable statement from the complainants that expresses in detail their version of the events that constitute the alleged professional misconduct or offense.

Assessment team members are chosen based on the nature of the case. The team typically consists of a psychiatrist, psychologist, internal medicine specialist, addiction medicine specialist, team director, and social worker. Each evaluator works with the patient separately and individually, completing an evaluation prior to team staffing. The patients are required to describe their version of events and background history to every team member. Team evaluators use an array of interview techniques, self-evaluation tests, written assignments, formal medical examination procedures, and psychological tests. The team then collectively constructs a dynamic causal hypothesis for the events that led to the complaints, determines whether professional impairment is currently present, suggests a diagnosis using criteria from the *DSM-IV*, and recommends courses of action.

The results of the team staffing are presented to the patient. The patient remains in the program long enough to receive feedback from team members' individual evaluations, and to develop an action plan to be implemented upon discharge from the assessment program. If it is anticipated that the patient will react to the information adversely, or that the meeting will constitute another intervention on the patient, the attending psychiatrist is asked to participate. The patient's responses and level of acceptance of the assessment results constitute another phase of the assessment process.

There are three possible outcomes to the assessment:

1. A personal and professional rehabilitation plan is developed in conjunction with concerned parties.
2. No clear picture emerges, or no conclusion is possible.
3. Professional rehabilitation is not feasible due to the nature of the problem or diagnosis.

THE PATIENTS

Between 1990 and 1993, 150 physicians, dentists, clergy, counselors, lawyers, and other professionals from thirty-three states and Canada were assessed because of allegations of professional sexual impropriety. Nearly all (93%) were referred because of a work-related problem; in the remaining 7 percent, a problem outside the workplace, such as arrest for exhibitionism, led the licensing body to be concerned about possible extension of the behavior to the workplace.

The characteristics of the persons assessed are shown in Table 1–1. Among the physicians, certain specialties were overrepresented relative to their numbers in the United States, whereas others were found in lesser numbers than expected. Internists and family practitioners were the largest groups represented, but that is because they constitute the largest physician groups in the United States. Psychiatrists, obstetrician-gynecologists, emergency room specialists, anesthesiologists, and urologists were overrepresented, suggesting that physicians in these specialities are at a higher risk for sexual exploitation. Pediatricians were underrepresented, implying they are a low-risk group.

Table 1–1. Demographics of Patients Assessed

Sex: 97% male

Age: 28–63 (median, 44)

Sexual preference: heterosexual (90%), homosexual (6%), bisexual (4%)

Race: Caucasian (85%), Asian (11%), Hispanic (2%), black (1%), and Native American (1%)

Profession: physicians (75%), dentists (5%), psychologists and social workers (6%), other medical personnel (nurse, physician assistant, physical therapist, premedical student) (4%), clergy (7%), and lawyers and administrators (3%)

With respect to marital status, 70 percent were married, 12 percent separated, 10 percent divorced, and 9 percent were single at the time of the initial assessment. However, because the patients were often experiencing a marital crisis at the time of the assessment, several of them separated or divorced in the following weeks and months.

Many professionals (30%) claimed no religion. For those who did, Protestants (41%) and Catholics (29%) constituted the largest groups, as expected, compared to their prevalence in the U.S. population at large. Although the actual numbers were small, it appears that Jewish (8%), Hindu (4%), and Greek Orthodox (4%) patients were overrepresented among the physicians assessed. It is interesting to speculate on the reasons for this. Within the United States, different cultural subgroups have different likelihoods of acquiring various addictions. For example, Jews have a lower prevalence of alcoholism than non-Jews (Patai and Patai 1989) and are underrepresented in the membership of Alcoholics Anonymous. On the other hand, it is our impression that Jews are overrepresented among the members of Gamblers Anonymous and in the twelve-step self-help programs dealing with sexual addiction. As we will see later, the majority of sexually exploitative professionals are sexually addicted; it may be that the probable increased vulnerability of Jewish professionals to sexual addiction was related to an increased vulnerability to sexual exploitation. Clearly this topic needs additional research.

The overrepresentation of Hindu and Greek Orthodox professionals has a different explanation. These helping professionals had come from other cultures, in which expectations of the relationship between the professional and patient differ from our own. In some cultures, for example, it may not be considered necessary to ask permission to touch the patient or to provide explanations for the touch, or it may be considered appropriate to touch patients in ways that are not acceptable to American patients. Opportunities for misunderstandings abound because of cultural dissonance and often because of a language barrier. Professionals from other cultures may need additional training in the standards of American professional–patient interactions.

STUDY RESULTS

The chief results of our review of professionals who were assessed because of allegations of sexual impropriety were:

1. Two-thirds of the professionals were guilty of sexual exploitation as defined by us.
2. There were four basic causes for sexual exploitation by professionals:
   a. inadequate education about appropriate sexual boundaries
   b. a life crisis
   c. addictive disorder
   d. Axis I or II psychopathology (other than addiction).
3. Addictive disorders are a prominent feature of the psychological makeup of professionals who have allegations of sexual impropriety—over half had an addictive sexual disorder, and a third were chemically dependent.
4. Only one-quarter of the group were found to be clearly unimpaired and safely able to return to professional practice immediately.

The study results are summarized in Table 1–2. Of the 150 professionals assessed, two-thirds were found to be sexually exploitative. Some cases were inconclusive because of incomplete information. For example, some professionals who were involved in legal proceedings were advised by their attorney to withhold information.

Table 1–2. Results of Assessment (N = 150)

	Yes	*No*	*Inconclusive*
Sexually exploitative	66%	27%	7%
Sexually addicted	54%	46%	
Chemically dependent	31%	69%	
Sexually addicted among all exploitative	66%	34%	
Sexually addicted among all non-exploitative	37%	63%	
Professionally impaired (potentially impaired, 10%)	58%	25%	7%
Victims of childhood abuse	80%	20%	

When assessed for the presence of addiction, half the total group were determined to be sexually addicted, and a third were chemically dependent. These figures refer to a combination of exploitative and nonexploitative professionals. Examined separately, the exploitative professionals had a higher prevalence of sexual addiction than the nonexploitative group but not a higher prevalence of chemical dependency. Two-thirds of the exploitative group were sexually addicted, compared with only one-third of those who were not exploitative. In contrast, the prevalence of chemical dependency was virtually identical in the sexually exploitative and nonexploitative groups.

Clinicians who work with chemically dependent clients have often observed a tendency for multiple addictions to coexist. In line with these observations, the sex addicts in the group were more likely to have concurrent chemical dependency (38% prevalence of chemical dependency) than were those who were not sexually addicted (21% prevalence of chemical dependency). Thus, the presence of sexual addiction increases the risk of chemical dependency.

These results tell us, first of all, that professionals who have allegations of sexual impropriety have a high prevalence of addictive disorders. They have a significant likelihood of being chemically dependent (31%), and an even greater likelihood of being sexually addicted (54%). Also, among those in whom exploitation is confirmed, the likelihood of chemical addiction is unchanged, but that of sexual addiction rises to 66 percent. Finally, the presence of sex addiction increases the likelihood of coexisting chemical dependency. *It is clear that all professionals accused of sexual impropriety need a thorough evaluation for possible addictions.* In addition to undergoing evaluation for psychiatric disorders, many chemical dependency treatment programs have clients complete screening tests for eating disorders, sexual disorders, compulsive gambling, and other addictive or compulsive behaviors. We highly recommend this.

One of the chief goals of assessment was to determine whether the person is professionally impaired. This was diagnosed in 58 percent of the patients. Another 10 percent were considered potentially impaired, meaning that on a day-to-day basis they were not impaired, but were at a significant risk that on any particular day, given the right set of circumstances, they might be impaired; such patients would therefore require treatment and then close supervision at work. Twenty-five percent of the patients were considered unimpaired, and in 7 percent the assessment was inconclusive. Without further evaluation, the "inconclusive" group could not be considered safe to return to practice. In other words, the assessment team could support return to work for only one-quarter of the group. Most of the others required treatment and then reevaluation.

Immediate postdischarge recommendations consisted of inpatient treatment for sexual disorders and/or chemical dependency in 53 percent of cases, outpatient psychotherapy in 30 percent, education about appropriate boundaries in 5 percent, no treatment in

2 percent, and no recommendation was possible in the 7 percent whose assessment was inconclusive.

For exploitative professionals who follow treatment recommendations and ultimately return to related work, typically a period of two years elapses between the time of assessment and return to practice. Although insufficient time has elapsed to complete a long-term follow-up of the professionals we assessed, later chapters will describe some cases with successful outcomes. Chapter 4 discusses the four bases for sexual exploitation that emerged from the assessment.

2

Development of Boundaries, Male Psychology, and the Genesis of Sexual Exploitation

> And if it is true that we acquired our knowledge before our birth, and lost it at the moment before our birth, but afterward, by the exercise of our senses upon sensible objects, recover the knowledge which we had once before, I suppose that what we call learning will be the recovery of our own knowledge.
>
> Plato, *Phaedo*

Sexual exploitation involves a violation of appropriate boundaries between the persons involved. In this chapter we explain how boundaries between people develop in childhood, and how distortions of healthy boundaries can ultimately lead to sexual exploitation. The following case vignette provides an example.

Bruce Kennedy, a 40-year-old minister, lost his job and his ordination as the result of a series of affairs with parishioners whom he was counseling.

When Bruce was 6 years old, his mother became ill and died and his father began drinking heavily. Bruce and his older sister were pretty much left to themselves. Bruce didn't know how to make friends. At night, when his father drove him home, he would stop at a bar and leave Bruce waiting in the truck, sometimes for up to three hours. Finally, at age 8 or 9, he began walking home instead of waiting, despite his fear of the dark. After that he didn't see much of his father.

By age 15 Bruce had a job at a filling station. Saturday nights would find him pumping gas and listening to the crowd at the nearby baseball stadium, wishing he could be there with some friends. His father got a driving-while-drunk citation nearly every month and his name was often on the front page of the paper. Bruce was embarrassed and ashamed, but learned to suppress his feelings. A youngster who had no parents to love and pay attention to him, he spent his lonely hours fantasizing himself the center of attention of a large group of people, admired and loved by them, nurturing them and being nurtured by them. A desire to become a clergyman began to grow in his soul.

After college Bruce worked in a hospital for several years, got married, and had two children. Realizing his long-held wish to be a minister, he entered a seminary and worked his way through by being a night watchman. His life became strictly study and work; contact with his family was minimal. Bruce's wife Barbara had to handle everything at home, and gradually became angrier and angrier. Bruce's pattern of isolation and loneliness continued.

When Bruce became minister to a small congregation, he found himself drawn to the counseling aspect. One day a woman came in for marriage counseling; her husband refused to participate. After several sessions, when she was particularly upset and crying, Bruce hugged her to comfort her. The touching rapidly escalated to a sexual affair.

After that there were others. With each one, when she first came in, Bruce was serious about wanting to help her, but soon gave up. Later he realized that most of the women had already sensed a neediness in him to which they responded. He knew his actions were wrong, but his values and morals somehow receded and his emotions took over. Each affair lasted until the woman decided to end it. If Bruce's wife suspected, she never said anything.

It wasn't that Bruce was oversexed—many times he and the current woman would just talk and hold each other. With each woman, there was a lot to talk about. He considered his relationship with each of the women to be a very intimate one. They were very interested in what he was doing and what he had to say, so he felt important.

For ten years Bruce had affairs with lonely women, until one woman told her best friend, who told her husband, who told the woman's husband who was on the church council. Bruce had to resign. After he left his job there was a hearing with the result that the church administrative body took his ordination from him. Barbara stood by him, but threatened to leave him should he ever have another affair. Bruce returned to his old hospital job, but found himself surrounded by needy women; within a year he was again having affairs.

In despair, Bruce began seeing a psychiatrist, who gave him a diagnosis of sexual disorder with addictive and exploitative features, as well as dependent personality traits. The abandonment and loneliness he had experienced in childhood had led to a belief that he had to earn love by caregiving behaviors. His need for connection and validation with women had resulted in his breaching significant boundaries between his professional and personal life and to exploitation of a number of parishioners entrusted to his care. Initially, therapy was accompanied by 12-step group support focused on containing his behavior; subsequently it focused on understanding how his childhood experiences had shaped his adult relationships. He received education on appropriate professional boundaries and was advised to pursue a career that did not involve counseling women.

The case of Bruce Kennedy illustrates the adverse consequences that a professional may experience when his dysfunctional childhood relationships result in a failure of development of appropriate boundaries. In Bruce's case, abandonment by both parents, social isolation, and the shame and embarrassment engendered by his father's reputation as the town drunk set up a pattern in which his need for connection led him to abandon his healing role as a minister and counselor and take advantage of needy parishioners.

Over 80 percent of the professionals we assessed were victims, as children or adolescents, of physical, emotional, or sexual abuse; emotional incest; or profound abandonment. Because of the cultural expectation that "real men should be tough," most never discuss these matters until they go through the transition from victim to victimizer, finding themselves in personal and professional crisis.

Professionals who have boundary problems are at risk of becoming sexually exploitative. To present a cogent discussion on male archetypal themes associated with sexual exploitation of power and position, let us review what is currently understood about boundary formation, the psychology of male growth and development, and the psychology associated with disorders in the process of male individuation and separation from family.

EARLY DEVELOPMENT AND THE DEVELOPMENT OF BOUNDARIES

Before birth, a baby is physically united with its mother. Starting with the birth event, the child goes through developmental stages of separation from her. At each stage the child defines appropriate physical, emotional, sexual, and spiritual boundaries between himself or herself and other people, and in the process develops a comfort zone and appropriate levels of interaction with others.

These stages were described by Margaret Mahler and colleagues (1975). As will be seen, each developmental stage results in a clearer definition of interpersonal boundaries. During the first few months of life, the baby cannot distinguish himself from others; it is as though he were still physically connected to the mother. Mahler calls this the *autistic* stage, from birth until the second month of life, during which the infant's task is to integrate himself physiologically into the world. During the *symbiotic* stage, ages 2 to 5 months, the infant's sensitivity to external stimulation increases, but he is still fused with mother and unable to distinguish "I" from "not I."

Mahler goes on to describe a third stage, *separation-individuation*, disidentification with the mother, when the infant comes to recognize that mother is a separate person. This critical stage consists of four phases. In the *differentiation* phase (age 6 to 9 months), the infant begins to explore both the mother and the nonmother worlds by using eyes, hands, mouth, and legs. In the *practicing* phase (10 to 16 months), the child's energy is directed outward. Early practicing begins when the child learns to crawl, and continues when he learns to walk. During the *rapprochement* phase (age 17 to 24 months) there are quick gains in acquisition of language skills and gender identification. Finally, individuality is established during the *consolidation* phase (24 to 36 months).

Each developmental stage results in a clearer definition of interpersonal boundaries. In describing the first stage of human development, which he describes as *trust versus mistrust*, Erik Erikson (1950) posits that the first and primary developmental task of emotional health in early life is the establishment of a basic sense of trust, which plays a critical role in one's perceptions of the world and the "others" in it.

Between ages 1½ to 3 years, children gradually develop a sense of separateness from others. They develop *ego boundaries*, which Fossum and Mason (1986) define as "the ego barrier that guards an individual's inner space, the very means he or she employs for screening and interpreting the outside world and for modulating and regulating his or her interactions with the world" (p. 63). They state that one cannot establish an identity without clearly defined boundaries.

MALE SEPARATION FROM MOTHER

Normal male sexual and emotional development is associated with disidentification with mother and counteridentification with father,

as described by Greenson (1968). A young boy's relationship with
mother must undergo fundamental change in childhood to establish an effective relationship with father and other male role models. He may then develop a secure self-concept as a male and a
sexual being.

The early mother–child relationship is most often the primary
determinant of the quality of all later experiences of love. The capacity for healthy human love is engendered by feelings of early
infantile security based on an adequate mother–son bond, and
having experienced the trust that our mothers, in the earliest stages
of our development, had our best interests at heart. The mother
establishes for her son the sense that, by extension, the world is a
welcoming, safe, and nurturing container in which he can grow.
A boy who learns that he can basically trust the world develops a
secure center of self that is capable of withstanding the normal vicissitudes of life. This perception leads to the judgment that life is
basically good and that there is a reasonable expectation that he
is going to get his needs met, both by others as well as through
his own resources. This also gives him confidence that he will not
be unnecessarily rejected. This judgment, in turn, results in self-
generated behavior that is directed toward getting his emotional
needs met.

This formative healthy attitude toward the world, oneself, and
others is an essential psychological paradigm for the capacity to love
as an adult. By internalizing his mother's love, a boy can use this
introject later in his capacity to both love others and empathetically
understand them. This internalized mother-love leads to what
Pedersen (1991) refers to as *primary narcissism*, a high regard for
oneself that is part of an enduring and healthy sense of self-worth
and self-love. Without this healthy love of oneself there is little hope
for a healthy love of the "other" as more than a reflection of a part
of ourselves or as a vestige of our early experience. Freud reduced
a man's wish for his mother to a sexual desire rooted in primitive
instinct. He did not acknowledge the relationship of this wish to
his early attachment to her or to his later need to achieve separation from her—while retaining some aspects of the feminine.

Disruptions or failures in this process lead to vulnerabilities and shortcomings expressed years later as personal insensitivity, ambivalence toward complex and sexual relationships, and misogyny (Stoller 1974).

OEDIPUS COMPLEX AND
PHYSICAL AND EMOTIONAL INCEST

Father and son may each feel envy toward the other based on their unfulfilled relationship with "Mom." Our fathers' emotional abandonment of us makes a sham out of our attempts at separation from mother. For if our fathers have not separated from their mothers—particularly if they have not retained a high positive regard for the feminine in themselves—how are we as sons and as future fathers going to acquire a positive masculine identity and retain a healthy integration of the feminine for ourselves? The psychological manifestation of this abandonment by the father is a man's *oedipal wound*. The Oedipus complex, as classically elucidated by Freud, underestimates the psychological suffering and damage men experience in being abandoned by their fathers. The present phallus-dominated image of masculinity is an immediate consequence of this woundedness. The fear of the father, the king, that his son will one day slay him makes sense in that our rage at father for abandoning us makes us want to kill him, both literally and symbolically. But instead we turn our rage against our brothers, against other men, against ourselves, and against the women we try to love. That is the effect of our oedipal wound.

Imagery of incestuous sexual relations occurs only in those children who have psychologically if not overtly incestuous parents. Incest is a symbolic psychological foundation of the individuation process and an integral part of it; it represents the natural endogenous function of kinship libido. At the same time, when unimpeded by family members' overt or psychological neurotic incestuous fixations, this endogenous tendency is counterbalanced by an equal exogenous tendency to move away from the family in the natural process of psychological differentiation.

The repudiation of the feminine has been problematic for many men, since the splitting from the anima causes them to develop a counterphobic stance about their emotional dependency, as well as an exaggerated and overly heroic relation to the world. The lack of separation from the mother coupled with abandonment from the father, as well as the splitting from the anima, lies at the base of the incest complex. A man in this untenable position is unable to form a stable relation with a woman; at the same time he cannot succeed in forming an identity with a protective father who understands and reinforces the importance of boundaries. Since he cannot adapt himself successfully to being either husband or father, he turns to the anima as daughter or child and attempts to incorporate her in a literal and physical way, which leads to overt or psychological incest. (Pedersen 1991).

SECONDARY NARCISSISM

A *secondary narcissism* may occur when the development of the primary love relationship (with mother) is incomplete or unsatisfactory. This manifests as exaggerated feelings of self-worth or self-importance, sometimes bordering on grandiosity. Mothers who have experienced narcissistic injuries themselves inevitably perpetuate these wounds on their sons. Unloved, rejected, and abused male children become instinctively abandoning, unloving, and abusive fathers to their own children. In this way the cycle is repeated. John Bowlby (1973), an English psychiatrist who has studied attachment and separation processes in children and the effects of abandonment by mothers, maintains that many defects traditionally explained by psychoanalytic theory can as well be traced to problems of bonding in early life experience. He speculates that many degrees of pathological detachment occur later in childhood and adulthood as defensive reactions designed to prevent the pain and humiliation of the possibility of future abandonment.

ROLE OF THE FATHER

The father is the second critical factor in determining a man's capacity to love. Pedersen (1991) feels that the mother is more instrumental in the development of a man's capacity to receive love, and the father is more instrumental in his capacity to give love. As mediator between the home and the world outside, the father sets objective standards and rules that his son is expected to meet. Sons learn early that they have to "perform" in order to keep their father's love flowing. This becomes a paradigm for how boys, and later men, relate to each other. The positive aspect of this as a model of relationship is that it may promote healthy competition and the development of competency. The negative side is that it fosters envy and rivalry between fathers and sons as well as between men. If the father is too authoritarian and doesn't create enough room for mistakes and experimentation, the model introduces a destructive potential that becomes manifest when love and power become fused.

A crucial developmental task for a young boy is to move from being a mother-identified to a father-identified son. The father's role is of critical importance here because his attitudes toward his wife, as well as his own mother, will shape what aspects of the mother his son feels safe to retain. In fact, the entire repertoire of the father's behavior toward all women is a determinant in shaping the quality of his son's relationships with women. If a father has been unable to integrate a healthy sense of the feminine in himself, he will unconsciously transmit his lack of regard for the feminine to his son. This can contribute to a fundamental ambivalence toward women: women are objects of desire but, at the same time, objects of derision. Further, this ambivalence is at the heart of what many men experience as the lack of a well-established inner life, which is so aptly symbolized by the mother principle.

EGO DEVELOPMENT AND THE SHADOW

In the psychological atmosphere created by parents, siblings, caregivers, and other important sources of love and approval, each child begins the necessary process of ego development. Ego development depends on our repressing what is "wrong" or "bad" in us, while we identify with what is perceived and reinforced as "good." As ego comes, so goes the shadow. What is disowned does not go away. It lives within us as an unconscious alter ego.

As the child's ego takes hold in awareness, a portion of it forms a mask, or *persona*, the face we exhibit to the world that portrays what we think and others think we are. The persona meets the demands of relating to our environment and culture, matching our ego-ideal to the expectations of the world in which we grew up. Underneath, the shadow does the work of containment. The entire process of ego and persona development is a natural response to our environment and is influenced by communication with our family, teachers, friends, and clergy through their approval and disapproval, acceptance and shame (Zweig and Abrams 1990).

MALE WOUNDING IN RESPONSE TO DEVELOPMENTAL FLAWS

Disruption or difficulty in any of the areas described above results in psychological wounding, unique to the individual man, which takes shape in response to developmental flaws. Once formed it has an autonomous life, and is carried into adolescence and adulthood. According to Hudson and Jacot (1991), its characteristics include the following:

- It is a central feature of male mental architecture.
- It is a source of unresolved tension.
- It exerts a formative influence on the imaginative needs that the male subsequently experiences.
- It imparts a characteristic bias to the expression of those needs.
- Its action is evident by a loose-knit group of telltale signs.
- Its influence can be temporarily overridden, but tends to stubbornly reassert itself over the long run.
- Its forms of expression, creative and destructive, are protean.

The wounding affects personal development and has profound influence on intellect, intimacy, and erotic imagination.

THE CONSEQUENCES OF INAPPROPRIATE BOUNDARIES: VICTIM TO VICTIMIZER

It seems counterintuitive that a person who devotes his life to helping others simultaneously chooses to exploit vulnerable patients. Schwartz (1995) writes, "One critical question is how individuals who seem to have integrity in most of their behavior, who sometimes are ministers, doctors, and others who devote themselves to caring for and helping others, are capable of extremely destructive behavior, seemingly without conscience" (p. 85). Based on his own work and that of Briere (1992) with sexual trauma victims and that of other clinicians who work with adolescent sex offenders, he describes how temporary relief from the stress of compartmentalized recall of toxic memories, affect, and impulse engendered by the sexual abuse is obtained by reenacting the trauma. That is, victimization of the child can eventually result in perpetration by the adult. The perpetration is preceded by failure to adhere to appropriate boundaries.

As stated earlier, over 80 percent of the sexually exploitative professionals we assessed were victims of physical, emotional, or sexual abuse; emotional incest; or profound abandonment as children or adolescents. Childhood wounds such as these may prevent the formation of healthy boundaries with others. Emotional wounds from parental neglect or abandonment, rigid family rules that prevent children from expressing themselves, physical or sexual abuse—all these result in the failure to develop healthy boundaries. Negative childhood experiences may prevent a person from getting close to others; conversely, fear of abandonment leads one to seek fusion with another person rather than healthy independence.

Persons with childhood wounds can grow up with rigid boundaries, as though they were surrounded by a wall, not letting anyone in, fearful of loving or depending on another person. Conversely, they may grow up with overly permeable boundaries, seeking fusion with another person at whatever cost, including the loss of self. Such people feel incomplete unless they are in an enmeshed relationship with another person.

Fossum and Mason (1986) use a zipper metaphor to describe the regulator of the boundary encompassing the intellectual, emotional, and physical self. Persons with self-respect have an internal zipper, so that they themselves decide when to let someone else in. On the other hand, individuals who experience childhood wounds and shut down emotionally develop shame-bound personalities with unclear boundaries. They have their metaphorical zippers on the outside, believing that they are regulated by others and the outside world. This leaves them vulnerable to exploitation by others.

According to Fossum and Mason (1986), "a characteristic of the external zipper is seen in what can appear to be a lack of common sense. Women or men with undefined boundaries often make poor judgments due to their incomplete interpreting screens, and are harshly judged as 'asking for trouble.' Undefined boundaries, with denial and repression, prevent clear access to one's sense of what is safe and what is harmful" (p. 72). This description can be seen to apply to the case of Bruce Kennedy, described at the beginning of the chapter. His need for connection with women clouded his judgment to the extent that he exploited those whom he counseled and derailed his career as a clergyman.

One currently popular line of thinking, "attachment theory," sets love against an evolutionary backdrop. British psychiatrist John Bowlby was struck by the similarities between human infants and children and their animal counterparts. Most baby animals need to form passionate attachments with their primary "caregiver" (usually the mother). Once an attachment has developed, they become depressed, desperate, and emotionally disturbed if they are separated from that caregiver. Seen from this perspective, most psychiatric illness is a form of mourning for lost or inadequate love. Bowlby found many links between disturbed adults and broken attachments in childhood. Falling in love, loving, and grieving loss are biologically necessary functions, elaborate emotional dramas that have evolved because they were strategic for survival. Diane Ackerman (1994) describes what happens when the attachment process goes awry. She concludes this discussion by saying:

Studies show that even one continuously sympathetic caregiver in childhood can make the difference between a seriously disturbed adult or someone who is nearly invincible. Childhood experiences do trigger, and sometimes garble or distort, the love relationships made later. But nothing is cast in stone. As the child grows, it forges new attachments and some of these may dilute bad childhood experiences. This is an important conclusion, because it suggests that abused children—who are, essentially, loving disabled—may still be helped later in life. [pp. 131, 136]

Professionals who have boundary problems are at risk of becoming sexually exploitative. Those with overly permeable boundaries have such a need for approval that they may engage in unethical behaviors to achieve this goal.

Dr. Ron Smith, for example, succumbed to a patient's suggestion that she would go to bed with him if he would supply her with narcotics. Doing so cost him his license on two counts—sexual exploitation of a patient, and inappropriate prescribing of opioid medications.

Dr. Margaret Bean-Bayog, an actual, prominent Boston psychiatrist, having unsuccessfully tried for years to conceive a baby, turned a suicidal young patient with borderline personality disorder into her symbolic child. Confusing her personal and professional roles, she infantilized her patient, calling him baby names and giving him gifts appropriate for a young child. She allowed him to photograph her in unprofessional comic poses. She participated in sexual fantasizing with him, leaving graphic written descriptions of sexual fantasies about him in her office, where he found them. After the young man committed suicide, the physician chose to give up her license permanently rather than face a humiliating public hearing. Women professionals who sexually exploit often do so out of role confusion arising from rescue fantasies.

Dr. Lawrence Wright, a family practitioner whose devotion to his patients often cost him time away from his own family, was so devastated when his wife left him after complaining for years of being neglected, that he became sexually involved with the first patient who tried to comfort him. The thought of being unattached was so unbearable that the opportunity to merge with another overcame his better judgment.

Professionals with overly rigid boundaries are also at risk of sexually exploiting. They may have suppressed their own needs for years, sublimating them by taking care of other people's problems. Imbued with a distrust of others, they maintain a false front of invulnerability. When they are finally overwhelmed by their unmet needs, they may tell themselves, "I deserve to take care of myself for once!" and allow themselves to become sexually involved with a patient.

Some professionals have such impermeable boundaries that empathy for others cannot penetrate. They exploit other people without compunction. These are sociopathic sex offenders who clearly need to be taught victim empathy. Even so, their prognosis for professional rehabilitation is poor.

As shown in this chapter, adverse childhood experiences can contribute to diverse psychopathology, including dependent personality disorder, antisocial personality disorder, and various sexual and addictive disorders. All may have as one end point the sexual exploitation of vulnerable persons.

3

Sexual Disorders and
Addictive Disease

It is important to sort out the differential diagnosis of the sexually exploitative professional. This chapter presents an overview of sexual disorders found in the *DSM-IV* and their relationship to addictive disease. Four brief vignettes illustrate the contexts in which sexual exploitation can occur:

> David Jones, a married, 45-year-old physician, lost his medical license after his physician partners learned he'd had affairs with several female patients and turned him in to his medical licensing board. Raised in a rigid religious home where sex was not discussed, David was a high achiever and good church member. Starting in his teens, he became progressively involved with pornography and masturbation, made uncomfortable sexual demands on his wife, began extramarital affairs, and finally had affairs with several patients, who he maintained were "mutually consenting adults." After undergoing assessment, he was advised to quit medical practice and obtain more therapy. Inpatient treatment for sex addiction broke through

his denial about the inappropriateness of his sexual involvement with patients. This was followed by outpatient treatment
using a cognitive-behavioral model useful for sex offenders, in
conjunction with attendance at a twelve-step program for sex
addicts. Eventually his license was restored, with the stipula-
tion that for five years he treat only men. David obtained a
job at a men's prison and continued working on his recovery.

Allen Peterson was a highly successful, married, 39-year-old solo
gynecologist whose life was permanently changed when a patient complained to the medical licensing board that Peterson
had had sex with her within days after performing a surgical
procedure on her. The licensing board was very lenient with
him, simply putting him on probation, but he knew something
was wrong and went to a counselor, who determined that he
was addicted to both sex and alcohol. He went through inpatient treatment for both addictions, became actively involved
for many years in twelve-step groups, and changed the nature
of his medical practice to a group setting where he would no
longer be isolated.

James Green, an unmarried, 35-year-old psychiatrist, lost his
license after having an affair with a patient. He was overwhelmed with guilt about the affair, knew it was wrong, but
could not stop. When the patient eventually filed a malpractice suit against him, his license was revoked and he was sent
for assessment. This showed that he was an active alcoholic as
well as obsessed with sex, pornography, masturbation, and
affairs, and in addition had a debilitating dependent personality disorder. He was advised to continue in treatment but to
leave psychiatry practice permanently. Years later, he remains
disabled professionally, although he is emotionally improved
and continues his addiction recovery.

Richard McNamara, a married, 32-year-old psychologist, lost his
license after the parents of a patient complained to his licensing board that he'd had sex with their teenage son, whom he

was treating. Multidisciplinary assessment confirmed that this was the first time he'd ever been sexually inappropriate with a patient, and showed no signs of an addictive or compulsive sexual disorder, but that he did have dependent personality disorder, which tended to result in unhealthy enmeshment with his patients. He underwent psychiatric treatment and changed careers to one that did not involve one-on-one patient contact.

As described in Chapter 1, one of the most important results of a multidisciplinary assessment of professionals who had allegations of sexual impropriety was the high prevalence of addictive disorders found: one-third of the sexually exploitative professionals were chemically dependent, and a full two-thirds had an addictive sexual disorder. The *Diagnostic and Statistical Manual of Mental Disorders* (1994) provides an extensive list of various sexual disorders, but addiction is not among them. Nonetheless, we have found the addiction model to be extremely useful in understanding and treating many sexually exploitative professionals; many persons have been able to return safely to professional practice after treatment, which viewed their behavior within an addiction framework.

To complicate the picture, an array of sexual disorders, addictive disease, and associated psychopathology often coexist when professional sexual misconduct or abuse occurs. This makes it difficult to determine if professional sexual exploitation is primary, or if the conduct is a symptom or complication of a psychiatric disorder, addiction, or medical illness, each requiring a different treatment approach. Not surprisingly, even the most experienced clinician may be somewhat confused at this point. This chapter reviews the various categories of sexual problems described in the *DSM-IV*, focusing on those that can be appropriately viewed within an addiction paradigm.

The *DSM-IV* groups mental disorders into sixteen major diagnostic classes, one of which is entitled "Sexual and Gender Identity Disorders." The sexual disorders are subdivided into three categories—sexual dysfunctions, paraphilias, and gender identity disorders—as well as a catchall category called "sexual disorder not otherwise specified" (NOS).

The sexual dysfunctions are characterized by disturbance in sexual desire and in the psychophysiological changes that constitute the sexual response cycle. These disturbances result in decreased sexual desire and/or performance and cause marked distress and interpersonal difficulty. Sexual dysfunctions include low sexual desire disorders (hypoactive sexual desire disorder and sexual aversion disorder), sexual arousal disorders (female sexual arousal disorder and male erectile disorder), orgasmic disorders (female orgasmic disorder, male orgasmic disorder, and premature ejaculation), and sexual pain disorders (dyspareunia, which is genital pain during intercourse, and vaginismus, which is severe vaginal spasm that causes pain for a woman and interferes with penetration). There is also a group of secondary and other sexual dysfunctions, which include sexual dysfunction due to a general medical condition, substance-induced sexual dysfunction, and a residual category, sexual dysfunction not otherwise specified (NOS).

The paraphilias are characterized by recurrent, intense sexual urges, fantasies, or behaviors that involve unusual objects, activities, or situations that occur over a period of at least six months and cause clinically significant distress or impairment in social, occupational, or other important areas of functioning. For some individuals, paraphilic fantasies or stimuli are obligatory for erotic arousal and are always included in sexual activity; in other cases, the paraphilic preferences occur only episodically, while at other times the person is able to function sexually without paraphilic fantasies or stimuli. In contrast to the dysfunctions, which are associated with decreased sexual functioning, the paraphilias are commonly associated with increased sexual activity, often with compulsive and/or impulsive features.

Paraphilic sexual activity revolves around fantasies, urges, or behaviors that are considered unusual or frankly deviant by society and generally involve (1) nonhuman objects or animals; (2) humiliation or suffering of the patient or partner; or (3) nonconsenting persons, including children. Even when such urges or fantasies are not acted upon, the level of distress may be sufficient to warrant a diagnosis; far more commonly, paraphiliacs have acted on their desires many times before a diagnosis is made (Morrison 1995).

Gender identity disorders (transsexualism), a third type of sexual disorder, are characterized by strong and persistent cross-gender identification accompanied by persistent discomfort with one's assigned sex. Transsexuals cross-dress to look like the other sex, not specifically for sexual stimulation. They may be sexually attracted to males, females, both, or neither.

Sexual disorder not otherwise specified (NOS) is included for coding disorders of sexual functioning that are not classifiable in any of the specific categories. One of the three examples given for this disorder is "Distress about a pattern of repeated sexual relationships involving a succession of lovers who are experienced by the individual only as things to be used" (*DSM-IV*, p. 638) This diagnosis has historically been the most common one to be used for patients identified as sexual addicts.

The descriptive term *sexual addiction* does not appear in the *DSM-IV.* Addiction professionals who encounter both compulsive and impulsive sexual acting-out behaviors in their patients have experienced paradigm and nomenclature communication difficulties with mental health professionals and managed care organizations that utilize *DSM* terminology and diagnostic criteria. This difficulty in communication has fueled skepticism among some psychiatrists and other mental health professionals regarding the case for including sexual addiction as a mental disorder. Since the concept of sexual addiction is integral to assessment of professional sexual misconduct, we present here an introduction to this model.

Stated briefly, a sex addict is a person who is obsessed with some type of sexual behavior, and whose behavior is compulsive and is continued despite adverse consequences. Diagnosis of sexual addiction can be extrapolated from the *DSM-IV* diagnosis of chemical dependency. According to this manual, three of seven criteria must be met for a diagnosis of psychoactive substance dependence (Table 3–1). Of the seven criteria, two refer to decreased control, two to continued use despite negative consequences, and one each to obsession with obtaining and using the substance, developing tolerance, and withdrawal symptoms. Five of the seven criteria refer to behaviors, and thus can logically be applied to other behaviors, such as sex or gambling.

Table 3–1. Diagnostic Criteria
for Substance Dependence

A maladaptive pattern of substance use, leading to clinically significant impairment or distress, as manifested by three (or more) of the following, occurring at any time in the same twelve-month period:

1. Tolerance, as defined by either of the following:
   a. A need for markedly increased amounts of the substance to achieve intoxication or desired effect.
   b. Markedly diminished effect with continued use of the same amount of the substance.

2. Withdrawal, as manifested by either of the following:
   a. The characteristic withdrawal syndrome for the substance.
   b. The same (or a closely related) substance is taken to relieve or avoid withdrawal symptoms.

3. The substance is often taken in larger amounts or over a longer period than was intended (loss of control).

4. There is a persistent desire or unsuccessful efforts to cut down or control substance use (loss of control).

5. A great deal of time is spent in activities necessary to obtain the substance, use the substance, or recover from its effects (preoccupation).

6. Important social, occupational, or recreational activities are given up or reduced because of substance use (continuation despite adverse consequences).

7. The substance use is continued despite knowledge of having a persistent or recurrent physical or psychological problem that is likely to have been caused or exacerbated by the substance (adverse consequences).

Any sexual behavior can be taken to excess or used addictively, including activities such as masturbation or sexual intercourse that are usually considered healthy or normal. The crucial issue is not the number of times the sexual behavior is carried out, but rather the consequences to the person's health, relationships, career, and legal status.

Carnes (1983) categorized addictive sexual behaviors into three levels. Level one contains behaviors that are considered normal, acceptable, or tolerable, such as masturbation, homosexual acts, and prostitution. Level two behaviors are clearly victimizing but are considered only nuisance crimes. These include unwanted touch (frotteurism), voyeurism, and exhibitionism. Level three behaviors are felonies, such as incest, child molestation, and rape. Addicts at levels two and three usually also exhibit level one compulsive sexual behaviors. Sex addicts generally engage in three compulsive behaviors. For example, a voyeur typically also uses masturbation and pornography. Thus, an adequate sexual history must address all potentially compulsive sexual behaviors.

More recently, Carnes (1991) developed a new typology of compulsive sexual behaviors. The range of fantasies, urges, and behaviors that can be considered addictive sexual disorders may be appreciated by reviewing in Table 3–2 the ten categories developed by Carnes. The categories are fantasy sex (compulsive masturbation and pornography); seductive role sex (extramarital heterosexual or homosexual affairs); anonymous sex; paying for sex (prostitutes, phone sex); receiving money or drugs for sex; voyeuristic sex (voyeurism, peep shows, strip shows); exhibitionism; intrusive sex (indecent liberties, rape, using position of power to exploit others); giving and receiving pain; and exploitative sex in which force or victim vulnerability (e.g., children, animals) is used to gain sexual access.

Table 3–2. Patterns and Themes of Sexual Addiction

1. *Fantasy sex*: compulsive masturbation, pornography.

2. *Seductive role sex*: seductive behavior for conquest; multiple relationships, affairs, and unsuccessful serial relationships.

3. *Anonymous sex*: engaging in sex with anonymous partners, having one-night stands.

4. *Paying for sex*: paying prostitutes for sex, paying for sexually explicit phone calls.

5. *Trading sex*: receiving money or drugs for sex or using sex as a business; highly correlated were swapping partners and using nudist clubs to find sex partners.

6. *Voyeuristic sex*: forms of visual sex, including pornography, window peeping, and secret observation; highly correlated with excessive masturbation, even to the point of injury.

7. *Exhibitionist sex*: exposing oneself in public places or from the home or car; wearing clothes designed to expose.

8. *Intrusive sex*: touching others without permission, using position or power (e.g., professional, religious) to sexually exploit another person; rape.

9. *Pain exchange*: causing or receiving pain to enhance sexual pleasure; use of dramatic roles, sexual aids, and animals were common themes.

10. *Exploitative sex*: use of force or partner vulnerability to gain sexual access.

Adapted from Carnes (1991), and used with permission.

Sexual improprieties and excesses that are considered addictive in nature can usually be classified into one of three major *DSM-IV* categories: paraphilia (either one or more specifically identified in the *DSM-IV* or paraphilia NOS), impulse control disorder NOS, or sexual disorder NOS. When the behavior does not fit easily into one of these categories, and is not considered a manifestation of some other *DSM-IV* Axis I diagnosis, then it can be diagnosed a work-related problem or a relational problem, utilizing a V code on Axis I.

Five of Carnes's categories can be readily identified in the *DSM-IV* as specific paraphilias. These include voyeuristic sex, exhibitionistic sex, pain exchange (sexual sadism, sexual masochism), as well as some types of intrusive sex (frotteurism) and exploitative

sex (pedophilia). Four of the remaining categories may be correlated with paraphilias: fantasy sex may be associated with paraphilic
urges not acted upon, anonymous sex may be used to permit expression of paraphilic behavior with decreased risk of consequences,
and paying for sex or trading sex are means by which a partner
who may permit paraphilic activity may be purchased.

Impulse-control disorders is another *DSM-IV* category that may
include sexual behaviors. Some authors have considered compulsive sexual behavior to be essentially an impulse-control disorder
(Barth and Kinder 1987). In our opinion, some cases of sexual
excess represent an impulse-control disorder, whereas most cases
are attributable to other *DSM* diagnoses that embrace the predomi-
nant compulsive features associated with sexual acting out. The
essential feature of impulse-control disorders is the failure to resist an impulse, drive, or temptation to perform an act that is harmful to the person or to others. The individual feels an increasing
sense of tension or arousal before committing the act and then
experiences pleasure, gratification, or relief associated with the
activity. Following the sexual acting out, there may or may not be
regret, self-reproach, or guilt.

The premier example of an impulse-control disorder listed in
the *DSM-IV* is pathological gambling. Although pathological gambling is classed as an impulse-control disorder, whereas substance
dependence is an addiction, the criteria are in fact very similar.
Both sets of criteria involve preoccupation, loss of control, continuation despite adverse consequences, development of tolerance with
prolonged use, and withdrawal symptoms when use is stopped.
Such overlap is also seen elsewhere in the *DSM-IV*, and accounts
for some of the difficulty and disagreements clinicians sometimes
have in diagnosing particular disorders.

As stated above, the *DSM-IV* category of sexual disorder NOS
specifically cites as an example the person who experiences a series of lovers only as things to be used. This category may therefore be correlated with addictive sexual behavior identified in the
Carnes categories of anonymous sex, paying for sex, trading sex,
and seductive-role sex.

What of other compulsive sexual behaviors that do not clearly fit into these categories, such as fantasy sex, seductive-role sex, and compulsive masturbation? If they cause distress to the person, they can be diagnosed as sexual disorder NOS, which is defined as "a sexual disturbance that does not meet the criteria for any specific Sexual Disorder and is neither a Sexual Dysfunction nor a Paraphilia" (*DSM-IV* p. 181). It is, however, instructional to see how such behaviors fit the diagnostic criteria for substance-related disorder as shown in Table 3–1.

There is significant overlap among *DSM-IV* diagnostic criteria, so it is possible for a single disorder to fit more than one diagnostic category. Some cases of compulsive sexual behavior may fit into the impulse-control disorder NOS and sexual disorder NOS, as well as fulfill the criteria for an addictive disorder. To remain within *DSM* terminology, Irons and Schneider (1994) code the results of Irons's assessments using paraphilia (either one or more specifically identified in the *DSM-IV*, or paraphilia NOS), impulse control disorder NOS, or sexual disorder NOS, but always with the inclusion of appropriate and relevant descriptors. Frequently addictive features are present. Other descriptors used include assaultive, compulsive, dissociative, ego dystonic, ego syntonic, exploitative, paraphilic, predatory, and sadistic. The use of descriptive features is especially helpful whenever an NOS diagnosis is utilized to bring clarity and precision to the diagnosis.

In addition to the categories thus far described, there are other *DSM* Axis I diagnoses associated with sexual excesses. These must be considered and ruled out before the patient can be labeled as having paraphilia, impulse-control disorder, sexual disorder NOS, or addictive disorder. The complete differential diagnosis is presented in Table 3–3; some of the disorders are discussed here.

Among the common diagnoses we have not yet discussed, manic-depressive illness, now called *bipolar affective disorder*, is frequently characterized by sexual excesses in the manic phase. According to the *DSM-IV* (1994, pp. 328–329), "The expansive quality of the mood is characterized by unceasing and indiscriminate enthusiasm for interpersonal, sexual, or occupational interactions. . . . The increase in goal-directed activity often involves excessive planning of, and excessive participation in, multiple activities (e.g., sexual . . .). Increased sexual drive, fantasies, and behavior are often present."

Table 3–3. Axis I Differential Diagnosis of Excessive Sexual Behaviors

Common:
  Paraphilias
  Sexual disorder NOS
  Impulse-control disorder NOS
  Bipolar affective disorder (type I or II)
  Cyclothymic disorder
  Posttraumatic stress disorder
  Adjustment disorder (disturbance of conduct)

Infrequent:
  Substance-induced anxiety disorder (obsessive-compulsive symptoms)
  Substance-induced mood disorder (manic features)
  Dissociative disorder
  Delusional disorder (erotomania)
  Obsessive-compulsive disorder
  Gender identity disorder
  Delirium, dementia, or other cognitive disorder

Cyclothymic disorder can be viewed as a scaled-down version of bipolar illness. Its essential feature is a chronic, fluctuating mood disturbance involving numerous periods of hypomanic symptoms and numerous periods of depressive symptoms. Hypersexuality may be seen during the hypomanic periods.

Substance-induced mood changes such as anxiety or euphoria may result in sexual preoccupation and activity, which can be then considered secondary to the substance use rather than an independent diagnosis. The challenge often is to sort out the role of the chemical use in the sexual compulsivity. For example, Washton (1989) reported that 70 percent of patients enrolled in his outpatient cocaine addiction treatment center exhibited sexual compulsivity. He found that some of these patients had no sexually addictive behaviors prior to cocaine use, and had no difficulty with sexual excess once cocaine use was stopped; clearly their sexual behaviors were secondary to cocaine abuse. Other patients, who showed evidence of an addictive sexual disorder antedating their cocaine use, clearly have two separate addictions. Still others found it difficult to stop their compulsive sexual behaviors after stopping cocaine use; they form a gray area, as their addictive sexual disorder may have originally been secondary to cocaine use, but seemed to have taken on a life of its own and needed to be treated in its own right.

Just as mood-alteration by chemicals can affect a person's sexuality, so can *cognitive disorders*. Dementia and delirium result in loss of the ability to judge the appropriateness of various behaviors; public masturbation, inappropriate sexual touching, and uninhibited language may be expressions of the altered social awareness.

Obsessive-compulsive disorder (OCD), which must be differentiated from a separate Axis II diagnosis of obsessive-compulsive personality disorder, has as its essential features

> recurrent obsessions or compulsions that are severe enough to be time consuming or cause marked distress or significant impairment. At some point during the course of the disorder, the person has recognized that the obsessions or compulsions are excessive or unreasonable. . . . The most common obsessions are repeated thoughts about contamination, repeated doubts . . . and sexual imagery (e.g., a recurrent pornographic image). . . . The individual with obsessions usually attempts to ignore or suppress such thoughts or impulses or to neutralize them with some other thought or action (i.e., compulsion). . . . Compulsions are repetitive behaviors (e.g., hand washing, ordering, checking) or mental acts the goal of which is to prevent or reduce anxiety or distress, not to provide pleasure or gratification. [*DSM-IV* pp. 417–418]

Some sexologists, such as Eli Coleman (1990), consider sexual compulsivity to be a variant of OCD. We agree that sexual obsessions may be an aspect of OCD. However, when compulsive sexual behavior is the primary disorder, the *DSM-IV* (pp. 417–418) specifically rules out the diagnosis of OCD:

> Some activities such as eating (e.g., Eating Disorders), sexual behavior (e.g., Paraphilias), gambling (e.g., Pathological Gambling), or substance use (e.g., Alcohol Dependence), when engaged in excessively, have been referred to as "compulsive." However, these activities are not considered to be compulsions as defined in this manual because the person usually derives pleasure from the activity and may wish to resist it only because of its deleterious consequences.

When sexual or seductive (romantic) behavior is the focus of obsessive mental activity, is neither acted upon nor produces gratification, and is causing significant distress, then it may meet the criteria for OCD. In our experience, such rare cases are associated with nonsexual behavioral manifestations of OCD.

Delusional disorder is the presence of one or more nonbizarre delusions that persist for at least a month. Apart from the direct impact of the delusion, the person's behavior appears normal and their psychosocial functioning is not markedly impaired. The delusion may be of being a prominent person or having a special relationship with such a person, or that the patient's spouse or lover is unfaithful, or that the patient is being conspired against, or that the patient has an infestation of insects on the skin or a bad odor. In the erotomanic type of delusional disorder (*DSM-IV* p. 197), "the central theme of the delusion is that another person is in love with the individual. The delusion often concerns idealized romantic love and spiritual union rather than sexual attraction. The person about whom this conviction is held is usually of higher status, but can be a complete stranger."

COMPLETING THE DIAGNOSIS OF
ADDICTIVE SEXUAL DISORDERS

In the differential diagnosis of sexual improprieties and excesses, Axis II characterologic disorders and traits are often contributory, or may be considered the primary etiology of paraphilic sexual behavior. For example, narcissistic personality disorder is associated with a person who has a grandiose sense of self-importance or a sense of entitlement; requires excessive admiration; believes he or she is special and unique, and can only be understood by other special people; is preoccupied with fantasies of unlimited success, power, brilliance, beauty, or ideal love; is interpersonally exploitative; lacks empathy; is often envious of others or believes others are envious of him; and shows arrogant, haughty behaviors or attitudes. Such an individual may readily view another person as an object to be used for one's own sexual pleasure. Although these personality characteristics may be seen as defects of character that can be resolved over time through unconditional surrender and dedication to a twelve-step program of recovery, some individuals are "unfortunates"—and "remain naturally incapable of grasping and developing a manner of living which demands rigorous honesty" (Alcoholics Anonymous 1976, p. 58). Such constitutional incapability is the essence of sexual excess that should be relegated to the primary diagnosis of a personality disorder.

CONCLUSION

The *DSM-IV* is our current standard for diagnostic criteria and for the classification of mental disorders that may entail out-of-control sexual thoughts and acting out. Rather than attempting to fit all cases into one model, addiction treatment professionals need to be knowledgeable about the spectrum of mental disorders that may be associated with sexual fantasy, urges, and behaviors. Even when the term *sexual addiction* is the most straightforward identification, and the one best received by the patient, the *DSM-IV* must be utilized for organizing, thinking about, and reporting the diagnosis.

Many sexually compulsive persons have seen multiple therapists without being able to effect any change in their behavior. The value of the addiction model for self-destructive sexual behaviors is that it suggests a new treatment approach. It is generally accepted that alcoholics are not often successfully treated by standard insight-oriented psychotherapy. The best results are obtained with confrontive, supportive, and educational group therapy in combination with mutual-help groups such as Alcoholics Anonymous. The same approach has helped thousands of persons in the past fifteen years to stop their sexual acting out and to turn their lives around. In the late 1970s, several mutual-help, twelve-step programs for sex addicts were founded and now claim thousands of members in the United States, Canada, and other countries. Programs for family members of sex addicts, similar to Al-Anon for family and friends of alcoholics, also exist.

Although the effects of sexual addiction on the addict and on the family parallel the effects of alcoholism and other drug dependencies, recovery from sexual addiction more closely resembles recovery from eating disorders. The goal is not abstinence, but rather the development of a healthy relationship—with food in the case of eating disorders, and sexuality in the case of sexual addiction. A brief abstinence period of one to three months is usually recommended at the beginning of recovery from sexual addiction. The great majority of sex addicts were sexually abused as children (Carnes 1991); they often require therapy to work through the psychological consequences of the abuse, and education about what constitutes healthy sexuality.

Sexual addiction often coexists with chemical dependency. Among recovering sex addicts, 29 percent were also recovering from chemical dependency, 38 percent were workaholics, 32 percent had an eating disorder, 13 percent characterized themselves as compulsive spenders, and 5 percent were compulsive gamblers. Only 17 percent believed they had no other addiction (Carnes 1991, Schneider and Schneider 1990). Sexual addiction is often an unrecognized cause of chemical relapse in recovering drug addicts. This is particularly true with cocaine addiction. In Washton's study (1989) about 70 percent of cocaine addicts entering an outpatient treatment program were found to be addicted to sex as well. Many patients had become trapped in a reciprocal-relapse pattern, in which compulsive sexual behavior precipitated relapse to cocaine use and vice versa.

Clinicians who treat addicts need to assess them for multiple addictions and recognize that an addict who stops one addictive behavior (such as excessive drinking or drug dependency) may substitute another addictive behavior (such as multiple affairs, over-eating, or increased smoking) as a means of mood alteration and escape. Not having addressed their fundamental addiction issues, they are then more vulnerable to relapse to the addiction that is ostensibly being treated.

4

The Sexually Exploitative Relationship

Sexual exploitation involves an interaction between two people. In this chapter we explain how relationships of unequal power differ from equal relationships, and how progressive boundary violations can lead to sexual exploitation.

> Transference love is, in many ways, medieval in structure. It's a love heightened by obstacles, taboos, and impossibilities, as was courtly love. That makes it all the more delectable. The therapist is like a knight who must prove his devotion by *not* lying down with his lady. Or rather, in effect, by lying down with her but not touching her. That was, after all, the final and truest test of a knight's love—if he could steal into his lady's chamber and climb into bed beside her, while her naked body appealed to all his normal male appetites, without laying a hand on her. In therapy, the patient lies down—literally or figuratively—and is more naked than naked, more exposed than nudity could ever reveal. The therapist proves his devotion by not responding sexually. His quest is to restore what has been lost or stolen from the castle of her self-regard. It is a difficult

task, which they both construe as a journey fraught with ob-
stacles and danger and strife. There are dragons to slay. There
are whirlwinds to tame. There are enemies without. There are
monsters within. [Ackerman 1994, p. 326]

When, after many years of service, the elderly Reverend
Christenson left the local church for a university position,
many in the congregation were not sorry to see him go. Under his dry, understated leadership style and with his highly
intellectual sermons, the church had lost many members, and
interest in church activities among the remaining members was
flagging. The arrival of the young, attractive, charismatic Reverend Jamison breathed new life into the congregation. His
sermons were vibrant and emotional, he instituted new programs of political activism, and he loved interacting with
people. "Jamie" had a knack for remembering people's names
and details about their lives, and his warm, welcoming manner encouraged those in need to come to him for counseling.

Over the next two years, membership in the congregation
doubled, and with it donations increased and more church
programs became possible. The church's sanctuary was refur-
bished and other buildings renovated. The poolside parties
that he and his wife hosted for the congregation several times
a year were well attended and served to increase Reverend
Jamison's popularity even further. Jamie was in constant demand for weddings, hospital visits, counseling, and just conversation.

What the congregation didn't know was that things were
not all well in Jamie's personal life. There had been friction
with his wife ever since she learned about an affair he'd had
out of town. Also, he suspected his adolescent daughter, his
middle child with whom he'd always had a special relationship,
was experimenting with drugs. His worries about her possible
drug use were tearing him up inside.

As his home life became more tense, Jamie found himself getting more and more of his self-esteem needs met

through his work. His increasing counseling duties and other responsibilities gave him legitimate reason to spend less and less time at home. Jamie was very aware of the exalted position in which his congregation held him, and he worked hard to maintain his public image. Very few people knew of his personal problems, of his sense of isolation at home, of his physical and emotional fatigue, of his worries about his vanishing youth as he passed his fortieth birthday.

One of those seeking counseling was Melinda, a 28-year-old mother of three small children whose alcoholic husband was becoming increasingly abusive. The warm, caring support Jamie gave her during counseling sessions over a several-month period was very helpful to Melinda. Jamie encouraged her involvement in church projects, where she soon made herself indispensable because of her desire to please and her willingness to undertake whatever was needed. The church projects also gave Melinda an opportunity to spend more time with Reverend Jamison. She felt valued and important and began to think she had the right to happiness in a relationship. Increasingly, she found herself comparing her uncaring husband with Jamie, with his warmth and understanding, and she wished that Jamie could replace her husband.

Jamie, meanwhile, was also doing some comparing. At home he regularly faced an angry wife who berated him for spending too much time at work and didn't appreciate all the efforts he was putting into helping so many people. Jamie's wife had long ago lost sexual interest in him. He was not only sexually frustrated, but he also felt devalued as a man and a husband. Melinda, on the other hand, needed him, looked up to him, and was thrilled at the attention he was giving her. She could see his inner pain over the many demands made on him, the role he had to constantly fulfill, the sense of responsibility for keeping the church going, the higher moral standards his congregation held him to, and his daughter's acting-out behavior. Melinda obviously worshipped him, and her attention assuaged his pain.

Gradually Jamie accorded Melinda special status as a counselee. He began scheduling her counseling sessions at the end of the day, so that he could give her extra time if needed. He could see how much she appreciated his hugs, and they became more frequent. Jamie found himself looking forward all day to his counseling session with Melinda.

It seemed inevitable that the counseling relationship gradually became more personal. When a sexual affair began, it seemed so right to both of them that they were sure it had to be God's will. Jamie's encouragement and support gave Melinda the strength to finally leave her abusive husband. Jamie was then faced with a choice—follow his heart and become Melinda's partner, or continue to make the best of his faltering marriage. Despite pangs of guilt, he left his wife. Jamie and Melinda both felt they had found true love, and, certain that others would understand, announced this publicly to the congregation in a letter asking for the membership's support.

Jamie and Melinda believed they were falling in love. Though both were aware that others would say they were committing adultery, they felt that their prior relationships had become intolerable, that they deserved better, and that their actions would be forgiven. What they did not acknowledge, or perhaps did not recognize, was that there was a larger ethical problem present—the exploitation by a person in a position of greater power of a person with lesser power. Relationships of unequal power include physician and patient, psychologist or therapist and client, clergyperson and congregant, professor (or teacher) and student, and parent and child. These are all relationships that are fiduciary, bounded, and involve sacred trust, relationships in which the person in greater power has an implied duty to act in the best interest of the other person. In all these relationships, the person in lesser power lacks the ability to truly consent to a sexual relationship. Accordingly, the person in greater power has the responsibility to act in the best interests of the other person, and these best interests do not include a sexual relationship.

SEXUAL EXPLOITATION:
A METAPHORICAL CLASSIFICATION

Sexual Exploitation as Incest

Why is a consensual sexual relationship between two adults of unequal power exploitative? One way to understand this is to look at the parallels between parent and children and professionals and client. Table 4–1, adapted from Blanchard (1991), makes this comparison of the father–daughter and professional–client relationship.

Table 4–1. Incest and Exploitative Professional Relationships

Father–Daughter	*Professional–Patient*
1. Age difference	1. Professional generally older
2. Intrinsic trust of father role	2. Intrinsic trust of professional
3. Greater power of father	3. Greater power of male in male-dominated culture
4. Authority of father	4. Authority of professional
5. Intellectual and educational superiority	5. Intellectual and educational superiority
6. Natural desire to obey and please father	6. Natural tendency to defer to and please professional
7. Psychological vulnerability of childhood	7. Psychological vulnerability of a client in crisis
8. A father's woundedness and vulnerability	8. A professional's woundedness and vulnerability

Adapted from Blanchard (1991), and used with permission.

As can be seen, the relationship between a professional and client greatly resembles that of a parent and child. In both cases the former has greater authority as well as intellectual and educational superiority, while the latter is more vulnerable, has a natural desire to please and obey, believes that the father/professional will act in her best interest rather than his own, and wants to heal her woundedness and vulnerability.

Another characteristic of the relationship of unequal power is that the person in greater power is generally in possession of more personal information about the other person than vice versa. For example, the patient will bare her body and express her innermost concerns about her physical and sexual health to her doctor, but not vice versa. The therapy client will bare her soul and reveal her deepest fears and weaknesses to a trusted counselor. In both cases, the client is allowing herself to be vulnerable because she believes that the other person is acting in her best interest.

Intimacy, Pseudointimacy, Transference, and Countertransference

Does intimacy exist in professional–client relationships? Schneider and Schneider (1990) defined intimacy as "the willingness to let our partner really know us, to exchange feelings and thoughts without fear of being judged or criticized. Intimacy requires vulnerability. Generally, we are willing to be vulnerable only if we trust our partner" (p. 78). When the client trusts the professional, becomes willing to be vulnerable, and lets the professional know her body and/or her innermost feelings and thoughts, she is likely to believe that intimacy exists between her and the professional. She will have warm feelings for the professional, and often a desire to increase the strength of their connection. Many patients wish to become friends with their therapist after the termination of counseling, precisely because of the intimate connection they already feel toward the professional. In addition, they mistake professional caring on the part of the therapist for personal friendship. They are confusing intimacy with engagement in the therapeutic covenant.

Many therapists with whom we spoke decline such overtures of friendship, not because they don't have warm feelings for the patient, but because they want to leave the door open for the possibility of a future professional relationship. In a relationship of peers, there are expectations on both sides, opportunities for disappointment, and the possibility of resentments developing. Once the character of the relationship changes in this direction, the door may close for either or both to feel comfortable in a future professional counseling relationship.

Is the professional–patient relationship really intimacy? In an intimate relationship, both people are vulnerable and reveal themselves. In contrast, in the ideal professional–client relationships, this is true only of the client. The professional may choose to reveal something of himself if he feels it will benefit the therapeutic relationship, but it is generally very little, and varies with the particular profession. Traditional psychotherapists, for example, reveal virtually nothing of themselves. At the other end of the continuum, addiction counselors who are recovering alcoholics or drug addicts find it useful to share some of their own addiction experience to show the client that "I was there too, and I truly understand." Physicians certainly do not expose their own bodies, whereas patients are routinely expected to do so when asked. The result is that the professional does not feel the same sense of vulnerability and intimacy toward the client as does the client toward the professional. When the professional does reciprocate the client's intimate feelings, as in the case of Rev. Jamison, there is danger, and a great risk of the loss of the therapeutic relationship. But when the professional–client relationship is appropriate, we may say that the client experiences pseudointimacy.

The classic experience that clients have had in their past that resembles the pseudointimacy of the professional–client relationship is their relationship with their parents. Melinda, for example, replicated with Rev. Jamison the relationship she had with her father in his last few years of life. It is easy for the client to develop an idealized, stereotyped image of the professional that is based on other relationships the client experienced. This process, called *transference*, results in the client's reacting to the *role* of the therapist rather to the individual behind the professional's role. The client then attributes to the professional those characteristics that the role represents, but that may not be true of the professional himself.

Melinda was responding in part to the admired father-figure leadership role that her minister represented, rather than to the person of Jamie himself. She viewed Rev. Jamison as a rescuer of a damsel in distress. Would she have responded the same way had Jamie been a postal worker or engineer she met in an office? Probably not.

Similarly, the professional may develop a stereotyped idealized image of the client, a process called *countertransference*. This is the tendency of the professional to repeat with the client aspects of previous important relationships. For example, a young doctor or therapist may idealize a patient who reminds him of a girl in high school he had a crush on but could never muster the courage to ask out. Or the professional may find herself sexually attracted to the client because he represents a person in need whom she can "save." For yet another professional, the client may represent the daughter he never had. Countertransference, like transference, is a normal phenomenon in relationships of unequal power, but is dangerous when denied, repressed, and not understood.

Why do some clients and professionals tend to sexualize or romanticize the transference and countertransference? The person's individual history and unique wounds may make him or her particularly vulnerable to this phenomenon. For example, a young girl may learn in high school that flirting is a short cut to getting her way. As she gets older, this pattern is reinforced and repeated, and becomes her usual way of dealing with men. If she was sexually abused in childhood, she may have been programmed early on to relate in this way.

As Ackerman (1994) writes,

> Each person is attracted over and over again to a predictable "type" of lover. Each has a habitual pattern of loving, and of losing. The men who have been left by a number of women have been left almost always in the same manner because of their character and of certain always identical reactions which can be calculated: each man has his own way of being betrayed. [p. 119]

The American Psychiatric Association's Ethics Committee wrote in 1989, "The necessary intensity of the therapeutic relationship may tend to activate sexual and other needs and fantasies on the part of both therapists and patients. . . . Sexual activity with a patient is unethical."

Commenting on the effects of transference and countertransference in physician–patient relationships, Nannette Gartrell and colleagues (1992) wrote,

> Because feelings of trust, dependency, gratitude, and intimacy are inherent in the physician–patient relationship, patients may find it difficult to decline sexual initiatives from their physicians. Some patients, because of their vulnerability, may interpret their physician's professional caring as personal intimacy and even initiate sexual advances. It is the physician's responsibility, however, to prevent the harm that may result from physician–patient sexual contact. [p. 142]

Attraction to Clients

It is natural for professionals to feel sexual attraction to particular clients for various reasons (Engel 1987, Pope et al. 1986). Probably every professional has experienced these feelings. The problem comes when these feelings are acted on, or even disclosed if the disclosure is designed to get a reaction that gratifies the professional. This dilemma was well described by psychiatrist Peter Rutter (1992) in his book, *Sex in the Forbidden Zone*. He explains the book's title as sexual behavior between a man and a woman who have a professional relationship based on trust, specifically when the man is the woman's doctor, psychotherapist, pastor, lawyer, teacher, or workplace mentor.

Rutter writes, "When a forbidden-zone relationship becomes erotically charged, several moments of decision inevitably occur that determine whether the sexuality will be contained psychologically or acted upon physically. Whenever a man relinquishes his sexual agenda toward his protégée in order to preserve her right to a non-sexual relationship, a healing moment occurs" (p. 215).

It is important for a professional to have a peer or supervisor with whom he or she can discuss feelings of attraction toward clients and get help in dealing with them so they are not acted on.

Acknowledging that sexual attraction to clients is normal, Pope and colleagues (1986) recommend that dealing with these feelings be part of the training program of psychologists. They write, "Educational programs must provide a safe environment in which therapists in training can acknowledge, explore, and discuss feelings of sexual attraction" (P. 157). Unfortunately, too many therapists in training have experienced sexual boundary violations in their relationships with their teachers. Pope and colleagues (1979) found that when educators engaged in sexual dual relationships with their students, those students were significantly more likely, when they became clinicians, to engage in sexual dual relationships with their clients. "Psychologists need to acknowledge that they may feel sexual attraction to their students as well as to their clients. They need to establish with clarity and maintain with consistency unambiguous ethical and professional standards regarding appropriate and inappropriate handling of these feelings" (p. 157).

Bennett and colleagues (1990), quoted in Corey and colleagues (1993), offer suggestions on how therapists can deal with powerful attraction to clients:

- Explore the reasons why you are attracted to a client. Ask if there is something about this person that meets one of your needs.
- Seek out an experienced colleague who might be able to help you decide on a course of action.
- Seek personal counseling, if necessary, to help you resolve your feelings about the client and to uncover the issues in your life that you may not be dealing with.
- If you are unable to resolve your feelings appropriately, terminate the professional relationship, and refer the client to another therapist. [p. 149]

Sexual Exploitation as Rape and Molestation

Thus far we have described one category of sexual exploitation— that which is analogous to incest. This category accounts for about two-thirds of cases of sexual exploitation by professionals. There are two other metaphorical categories of sexual exploitation—rape and molestation. They are compared in Table 4–2.

TABLE 4–2. Metaphorical Classification of Sexual Exploitation

	Incest	*Rape*	*Molestation*
Emotional dependency of victim	Yes	Perhaps	No
Transference	Yes, positive	Perhaps	No
Countertransference	Yes, positive	Negative	None or negative
Use of force	Covert	Overt	Not necessary
Coercion	Covert, indirect, gradual	Direct and immediate	When used, to get victim to vulnerable place
Ability of victim to resist, defend self against assault	Moderate	Moderate to low	Little if any
Risk of physical harm	Low	High	Moderate
Modus operandi themes	Seduction	Power, control over the weak, sadomasochism	Find the unprotected, grooming of children
Prevalence among sexually exploitative professionals	67%	25%	8%

About one-quarter of exploitative professionals seek power and have a desire for control. Their behavior can be considered a form of rape. They sexually exploit patients through physical force, intimidation, blackmail, or direct coercion. The risk of physical harm to the patient or client is high. They are usually not addicts, but rather have psychiatric diagnoses such as narcissistic, sociopathic, borderline, or schizoid personality disorders.

A few cases of sexual exploitation are analogous to molestation, because the offenders abuse helpless, defenseless people such
as those with physical or mental handicaps, patients under the influence of alcohol or sedative drugs, or patients who are under
anesthesia. The victim has little if any ability to resist the assault at
the time, so that physical force is not necessary. These offenders,
too, generally have primary psychiatric diagnoses other than addiction. Sexually exploitative professionals who offend on the basis of
rape or molestation themes generally have a poorer prognosis for
rehabilitation than do those who metaphorically commit incest with
their patients or clients.

THE ROLE OF SEDUCTION IN
SEXUAL EXPLOITATION

Most professionals are able to recall particular clients who appeared
interested in more than a professional–client relationship. Many
professionals can identify a few occasions when their feelings toward a particular client extended beyond professional concerns.
Who are these seductive clients, and how do they consciously or
unconsciously invoke emotional responses and personal reactions
from the professional? Most of the information we have about clients who have appeared seductive to their professionals comes from
studies of those who have reported professional exploitation, and
are the identified victims. Studies of female victims of exploitative
male mental health professionals have provided a profile that includes a number of common characteristics. Gutheil (1991) identified these as vulnerability, borderline dynamics, role confusion,
covert hostility, and special status.

Vulnerability

Clients who are vulnerable to sexual exploitation are often those
who have experienced some developmental trauma such as physical or sexual abuse or emotional incest. Sexually abused children
commonly present in adulthood with a mixture of psychosocial
problems, somatic symptoms, physical problems such as sexually

transmitted diseases, eating disorders, relationship problems, or sexual disorders. For children who were chosen by a parent for affirmation and emotional fulfillment by being placed in the role of surrogate spouse, this exploitation of power represents an abrogation of traditional roles and responsibilities. Adult children of emotional incest often have difficulties in relationships involving a power disparity.

Some clients were emotionally manipulated and even sexually exploited in previous relationships with teachers, counselors, clergy, or other professionals in a position of trust. The residual scars from such ethical violations often persist and affect future relationships with professionals.

Other vulnerable clients are those who are in emotional crisis. A life-changing event such as separation from the spouse or the recent death of a parent may leave them emotionally vulnerable and prone to seeking solace and comfort from someone they admire and trust. Two other contributors to client vulnerability are the presence of alcoholism or other substance abuse or addictive disorder, and the existence of anxiety, depression, or other mental disorder.

Borderline Dynamics

As a result of past physical, emotional, or sexual abuse, clients may develop specific behavior patterns that can be invoked whenever they find themselves on the bottom end of a relationship where there is a disparity in power, position, or authority. A history of neglect or rejection, rather than abuse, may activate this pattern, which is often directed only at individuals of the same sex as the one who previously hurt them. These behavioral patterns, termed borderline dynamics, should not be equated with borderline personality disorder, though there are common features. Such clients often feel numbness or emptiness in their current life, and seek affect-intensifying experiences to help them feel more real and alive. They often harbor fantasies of being rescued by a prince or princess who will make their dreams come true. They may impulsively and unpredictably pursue objects of fantasy and desire, with potentially disastrous consequences in a pattern of *repetition compulsion*, a term coined by Freud to define the tendency of individuals to repeat past behavior despite the suffering experienced with it, in an attempt to gain mastery over the initial trauma.

Role Confusion

Clients who appear seductive to the professional commonly are confused about appropriate professional and patient roles. They may interpret a hug given by the professional to express comfort or support as a sign of erotic or romantic interest. The physical contact required to complete a physical examination or diagnostic procedure by a physician may feel erotic rather than diagnostic to the patient. The client may have distorted expectations of the interaction with the professional and a desire to comfort and please him or her. The client may leave the visit unsure of whether anything inappropriate has taken place, yet feel uncomfortable and upset about the feelings the visit engendered in her.

Covert Hostility

Many clients are uncomfortable with the client role, resenting the professional's power, expertise, and knowledge. Especially when the professional does not fulfill the client's expectations for cure or improvement, the professional may become the recipient of the client's negative transference—unresolved anger toward an authority figure. The use of seduction to achieve a special relationship with the professional is one way for the client to gain power in the relationship.

Special Status

When a client receives special treatment in the form of reduced fees, longer appointments, home visits or after-hours appointments, exchange of gifts, or frequent telephone calls, the client may become confident that the professional views him or her as special.

This fosters greater idealization and projection in the relationship, and may in retrospect be interpreted by one or both parties as seduction.

Either the professional or the client can bring eroticized or romanticized thoughts, feelings, or gestures, into the professional–client relationship. However, for seduction to proceed to romantic or sexual involvement, both parties must consciously or unconsciously participate in an interactive process. This means that even if the client is seductive, the professional has the opportunity, and the responsibility, to prevent the relationship from entering the forbidden zone.

WHO GETS EXPLOITED?

Not all clients have an equal likelihood of finding themselves enmeshed in a sexual relationship with a helping professional. Clients who are seductive are, of course, at increased risk. Not surprisingly, the same factors that lead a client to become seductive are also risk factors for being sexually exploited. These include:

1. Domestic violence in the client's family of origin.
2. Childhood physical, emotional, and sexual abuse.
3. Emotional incest syndrome.
4. Existing psychiatric disorder.
5. Psychotropic medications.
6. Abuse in adolescence or young adulthood by another person in power.
7. Substance-related disorder or eating disorder.

CONSEQUENCES OF SEXUAL EXPLOITATION

Rev. Jamison and Melinda, whose story we presented at the beginning of the chapter, wrote a letter to the congregation of his church, requesting support for their new relationship. To their surprise, the congregation was not only unsympathetic, but a majority of the members were downright hostile. Most members felt betrayed by the reverend's adulterous behavior, though only a few recognized the sexual exploitation involved. The congregation split into two armed camps, pro-Jamie and against-Jamie. After several bitter congregational meetings, Jamie was fired and Melinda was ostracized. Investigation by the church's national governing body resulted in Jamie losing his ministerial privileges. The church experienced a major loss of membership and a spiritual crisis from which it took years to recover.

During the months until the resolution of the case, Jamie and Melinda, having lost their friends and social support system, drew closer together in their isolation. At the end of the year they moved to another state where Jamie, at age 40, began training for a new career.

Melinda continued to believe that meeting Jamie was the best thing that had ever happened to her; in a sense, Jamie's sacrifice made her feel like Wallis Simpson, the woman for whom King Edward VIII gave up the British throne in 1936. She was hesitant, however, to describe to new acquaintances the circumstances under which she and Jamie met, and regretted the loss of her church relationships.

Jamie's three children took his divorce and departure very hard. His middle daughter, in particular, was very angry, cut off all communication with him, and intensified her drug abuse. The other children phoned him frequently and told him how much they missed him. While doing his best to become a father figure in the life of Melinda's 6-year-old son, Jamie experienced recurrent pangs of guilt over his absence from his own children's lives. At times he found himself resenting Melinda.

EFFECT ON VICTIMS

One of the myths of professional sexual exploitation is that many of the victims are not hurt. Initially the person with less power often does not feel exploited, but as we saw in the above vignette, there may be other victims. Moreover, although relationships such as Jamie and Melinda's usually begin auspiciously, they tend to deteriorate over time. The power inequity that characterizes the early stages persists, and the decision to end the relationship usually comes from the person with greater power. The result is not just the pain of the ending of an intimate relationship. Rather, the former client feels exploited, and develops a predictable set of feelings that are often destructive of the person's self-esteem and willingness to trust others, especially professionals (Pope 1988). As a result of the unwanted ending of a relationship of unequal power, clients can experience the following:

1. Decreased self-esteem.
2. Impaired ability to trust. They mistrust themselves for having developed a trust for the physician. They mistrust others, especially professionals.
3. Deep ambivalence about the exploitative professional. They still have positive feelings about the value of the therapy and about the therapist.
4. Guilt and self-blame:
   a. Guilt for getting involved sexually with the therapist.
   b. Guilt for continuing the involvement.
   c. Guilt for believing they meant something special to the therapist.
   d. Guilt for not telling anyone sooner.
5. Sense of emptiness and isolation—as if only the professional could fill the emptiness. Part of this is loss of the "inner therapist"—the helpful internalized figure of the therapist with whom the patient can converse long after therapy has stopped.
6. Sexual confusion and sexual trauma. For some, any sexual activity may bring back traumatic memories. Others may be trapped in ritualistic, compulsive, or self-destructive sexual encounters and activities.
7. Depression or anxiety, and increased suicidal risk.
8. Suppressed rage, or overt anger at being exploited. There may be unresolved anger and a desire for revenge or retaliation.
9. Cognitive dysfunction, such as difficulty concentrating and intrusive thoughts.

Clients are often reluctant to report physicians or therapists, and typically wait years to do so. They can hardly believe what happened; they often blame themselves; they fear the professional's wrath; they may still care about the professional and fear ruining his practice; and they think no one will believe them anyway, especially if they have emotional problems or are alcoholic. At times they may find themselves pathologized by the system, as the professional attempts to defend himself against charges of exploitation by claiming that the client's psychiatric disorder or chemical dependency made her imagine the whole thing.

Two case histories from our practices illustrate the points we have made in this section.

Joan, aged 40, came to see her physician while in acute emotional crisis. Underweight and appearing ill at the time of the latest visit, Joan had a history of bulimia, depression, and sexual abuse, and until three years earlier had been getting counseling from a male therapist. She related that she had gotten into a sexual relationship with him and had become very dependent on him emotionally over a several-month period. One day the therapist unexpectedly terminated the sexual and the counseling relationship. He told her he had recognized that his pattern of sexual involvement with clients was addictive, was getting help for himself, and could no longer have any contact with her. After a suicide attempt and hospitalization, she gradually improved, but her emotional health remained very fragile and she was unwilling to obtain additional psychotherapy. Her self-esteem remained low, and she still thought a great deal about the exploitative therapist, her feelings alternating between longing for him and great anger. She felt there had been no closure between them and he was still a part of her life. The current emotional crisis resulted from a chance meeting with the man at a public lecture. When he had walked right past her without acknowledging her presence, she felt rejected all over again.

Joan's physician contacted the counselor and suggested

a supervised meeting between him and Joan to allow Joan to express her feelings and to obtain closure. Although he stated he felt terrible about his role in Joan's current emotional difficulties, the counselor was unwilling to have any contact with her under any circumstances. He stated she had borderline personality disorder and he was afraid that if they began a dialogue she would threaten him or his family, begin stalking him, or attempt to reignite their relationship. Joan finally agreed to begin seeing a new therapist for long-term psychotherapy.

Susan, aged 50, was in recovery from alcoholism for five years when she told her primary physician that she had been sexually assaulted by a gynecologist during a medical examination some eight years previously. She had never told anyone about it because she had been drinking heavily in those days, and she had assumed that no one would believe her. Besides, she wondered if she had somehow brought the rape on herself. Currently in counseling, she was only now dealing with this experience and wondered what, if anything, she should do about it. Both the physician and the therapist encouraged her to report the event to the state medical licensing board, even though the offending physician had since left town. It was explained to her that even though it might be too late to take legal action against him now, her report might help another victim if there were a new complaint against him. After working through residual feelings of guilt and disloyalty, she filed the complaint, and said she finally felt a sense of closure about the experience.

Adult relationships of unequal power can often be viewed symbolically as parent–child relationships rather than a relationship of peers. As in parent–child relationships, the potential for exploitation exists, and can often be masked as caring behaviors. The right course of action is not always clear, and subtle boundary violations can end as sexual exploitation, even when the intentions of the person in power were initially to help the patient.

The risks of sliding into exploitative actions are increased when the professional's training has not included education on ethical boundaries, and particularly if the therapist, clergyman, or physician has himself been the victim of sexual exploitation during training. The history of psychiatry is replete with sexual boundary violations perpetrated on vulnerable patients by the giants of the field; Carl Jung, Otto Rank, August Aichhorn, Karen Horney, and Frieda Fromm-Reichmann all had sexual relations with patients (Gutheil and Gabbard 1993). Freud encouraged one of his patients, a young psychoanalyst named Horace Frink, to divorce his wife and marry a patient with whom he had fallen in love. According to Gutheil and Gabbard (1993), Frink followed Freud's advice, and subsequently experienced deterioration in both his mental health and his marriage to the patient.

Even in the best-case scenario, when both parties believe that they are making a free choice to get sexually involved, unconscious forces are influencing that choice and making it likely that sooner or later one or both will be adversely affected. Long after the professional relationship has terminated, these same forces may still be in place. This has led to some controversy over the appropriateness of sexual involvement with former patients or clients (see Chapter 5).

5

When Is a Professional Sexually Exploitative? Gray Areas

Dr. Donald Prentice, a 50-year-old widower, was a clinical professor at the local medical school. He had two responsibilities at the school—he lectured a few times a year on his specialty, hematology, and he supervised students who rotated for six or twelve weeks through his clinic in order to learn about hematology. After attending one of his lectures, Jessica Bayless, a 35-year-old divorced first-year medical student, found herself admiring Dr. Prentice's teaching skills and his enthusiasm about his work. She asked Dr. Prentice to let her spend her one free afternoon each week working with him at his clinic. The more she saw of him, the more she admired him, and soon her admiration became more personal. Dr. Prentice found himself responding, and eventually they began a romantic and sexual relationship. Dr. Prentice encouraged Jessica in her medical career and she began to consider him her mentor.

A year later, Jessica chose to do a six-week elective rotation with Dr. Prentice. A committed and enthusiastic student, she worked very hard and received an excellent evaluation from

Dr. Prentice. Later he wrote her a first-rate recommendation
for her internship. Their sexual relationship ended after she
graduated from medical school and moved away. Subsequently
each of them remarried, but both remembered fondly their
time together.

When this couple first began a romantic relationship, they
were both unmarried adults with a minimal power differential. Dr.
Prentice was not acting in any official supervisory capacity over
Jessica; he provided her with a learning opportunity in his clinic,
but was not grading her. Only after she signed up to do an elective clinical rotation with him was he in a position to influence her
grades and therefore could be said to be sexually exploiting her.
On the other hand, at this point he was also vulnerable to potential charges by Jessica of sexual harassment of a student, and in
addition Jessica was in a position to exploit their sexual relationship by soliciting potentially undeserved good grades and recommendations.

Whether this scenario (and others to be discussed in this chapter) involves sexual exploitation remains controversial in some cases,
whereas consensus is gradually developing in others. In some cases,
such as employer and employee, current law now defines the problem as sexual harassment. In others, rules and regulations rather
than law defines the relationships, as in the case of professors and
their own students.

As discussed in Chapter 4, one type of sexual relationship
clearly considered unethical is that between a helping professional
and his or her current patient or client. The American Medical
Association, American Psychiatric Association, American Psychological Association, and other related professional organizations all
agree that a sexual relationship between a practitioner and a current patient or client is unethical. As summarized by Gabbard and
Nadelson (1995), there are three reasons such a relationship is
unethical:

1. It is a breach of the trust that is fundamental in a fiduciary
   relationship.

2. It calls into question the professional's capacity for objective professional judgment.
3. Because of the transference that the patient typically develops, the professional may be viewed as an all-knowing parent, and the patient turns over a great deal of power to him.

These dynamics are of greatest concern when the two people have a long-standing relationship and particularly when the patient's emotional state is the subject of the treatment. Gabbard and Nadelson's points refer specifically to a *current* relationship between a medical professional and the client or patient.

There are obvious and unquestionable scenarios of professional sexual misconduct and offense wherein the exploitation of power and position is readily apparent and the damage and adverse effects on the patient or client are salient. In our experience, there are also many scenarios of alleged professional misconduct or impropriety that are not so easily classified as exploitative and in which adverse effects on the "victim" are so difficult to define that there is no ethical or legal mandate to punish the "offender" or rescue the victim from the situation. Sexual and romantic relationships commonly develop between two people of different ages and in disparate cultural and socioeconomic classes. It is not realistic to assume that they do not harbor some power differential. Yet we would not consider restricting couples in these categories, unless one or both parties were minors or in some other way disabled or impaired in their ability to enter into a consensual relationship.

However, we are dealing here with scenarios where one party is acting in a professional capacity and the other is in one way or another paying for his expertise. Within this subset of relationships there remain a number of scenarios in which exploitation is considered controversial and where experts do not agree. These gray areas, in which the boundary between ethical and unethical, legal and illegal conduct, is not a line but rather at present a demilitarized zone, include the following:

- sexual or romantic relationship with a former patient or client

- sexual or romantic relationship between people who have had a very brief professional relationship
- intimate relationship between a professional and the family member of a patient or client, such as parent or child
- intimate relationship between a minister and member of the congregation in which limited pastoral counseling or personal services have been given
- intimate relationship between an attorney and a recent or former client
- intimate relationship between an adult student and the teacher or professor
- professional relationship between two people who previously had an intimate personal relationship.

A discussion of these situations will be followed by some guidelines to assist the clinician in maintaining appropriate boundaries and avoiding harm to the client.

CASE STUDIES

Sexual or Romantic Relationship with a Former Patient or Client

Dr. John Samuels, an unmarried, 35-year-old clinical psychologist, does intensive, long-term psychotherapy with Lillian Barnes, a 37-year-old divorced woman, whom he gets to know very well during a three-year period. Transference and nonsexualized countertransference lead to strong positive feelings on both sides, which are kept in check during the therapy. The feelings are discussed in therapy, and Dr. Samuels explains to Lillian that these feelings are a reflection of their therapy relationship, and not to be acted on. His feelings for her persist after the termination of therapy. He phones her occasionally to find out how she is doing. This leads to several informal meetings beginning twelve months after official termination and eventually a romantic/sexual relationship evolves, which began about twenty-five months after the official termination of therapy.

Intimate Relationship Between a Minister and a Member of His Congregation in Which Limited Pastoral Counseling or Personal Services Have Been Given

Reverend Bob Sanderson, a widowed, 65-year-old clergyman, has for fifteen years befriended and at times counseled a member of his congregation, Mrs. Atkins, now 62, whom he has gotten to know very well and has found attractive. His behavior toward her has always been very professional. Mr. Atkins dies after a long illness, and Rev. Sanderson finds himself spending more and more time with Mrs. Atkins and develops personal feelings for her. He continues to comfort her in her bereavement and gradually their relationship becomes a romantic one, which includes the expression of physical intimacy but no genital touching. He recognizes that maintaining a dual relationship with her, as both spiritual advisor and romantic partner, is not desirable. After several months, Rev. Sanderson suggests that Mrs. Atkins transfer to a different congregation so that he will feel more comfortable pursuing a personal relationship with her. Eventually they begin to attend social and church events together. Their relationship progresses into one that includes sexuality and overnight stays at each other's houses. Reverend Sanderson's church council questions his professional conduct and ethics, even though he has not specifically broken established national church policies.

Discussion

Sexual relationships within ongoing professional relationships are generally considered unethical. However, the ethical nature of sexual contact after termination of the professional relationship is a subject of much debate. With regard to physicians, Gartrell and colleagues (1992) suggest two guidelines:

1. The professional relationship must have been terminated with no intent of future sexual involvement or a continuing social relationship. In the two years after termination,

there have been no office visits, no prescriptions written, no telephone consultations, and no return appointment reminder postcards. The key issue is not time, but a discontinuous relationship.

2. The physician and former patient meet again in a context entirely unrelated to the previous professional encounter.

As to the duration of the waiting period, Linda Jorgenson, an attorney who specializes in ethical issues, has suggested that a three- to six-month waiting period after termination of a doctor–patient relationship is more reasonable than two years (Applebaum et al. 1994).

This issue was also addressed in a position paper, "Sexual Misconduct in the Practice of Medicine," published in 1991 by the Council on Ethical and Judicial Affairs of the American Medical Association. Its position is as follows:

> Sexual contact between a physician and a patient with whom professional relations had been terminated would be unethical if the sexual contact occurred as a result of the use or exploitation of trust, knowledge, influence, or emotions derived from the former professional relationship. The ethical propriety of a sexual relationship between a physician and a former patient, then, may depend substantially on the nature and context of the former relationship. . . . The length of the former professional relationship, the extent to which the patient has confided personal or private information to the physician, the nature of the patient's medical problem, and the degree of emotional dependence that the patient has on the physician, all may contribute to the intimacy of the relationship. [p. 2743]

The emotional involvement of a helping professional and a client or patient may vary widely, ranging from minimal involvement when there has been only a brief professional encounter in an urgent care setting, to an ongoing long-term relationship focused on the patient's vulnerable psychological state. Relationships between mental health professionals and their clients tend to fall on one end of this spectrum, an end where there is potential for more harm because of greater emotional involvement and greater disclosure of personal information that may be exploited. For these reasons, sexual relationships between patients and psychiatrists or psychotherapists are particularly discouraged by the Council on Ethical and Judicial Affairs (1991): "In most patient–psychiatrist relationships, the intense and emotional nature of treatment makes it difficult for a romantic relationship between a psychiatrist and a former patient not to be affected by the previous professional relationship" (p. 2743). This viewpoint is in agreement with that of the American Psychiatric Association, which states (1989) that "sexual involvement with one's former patients generally exploits emotions deriving from treatment and is therefore almost always unethical."

Consensus has gradually evolved among psychologists and psychiatrists that sexual involvement between psychotherapists and former clients or patients is unethical, no matter how much time has elapsed. In the case of psychologist Dr. Samuels and his long-term client Mrs. Barnes, they have spent years in a relationship of unequal power, in a symbolic parent–child relationship as explained in Chapter 4, and it is unlikely that they will be able to convert this to a relationship of peers. Dr. Samuels is in possession of a great deal more knowledge of Mrs. Barnes's psyche than she has of his, so that he still has significantly greater power in the relationship. At some later time she may resent this power disparity and feel exploited.

Moreover, by converting the relationship from therapeutic to romantic, Dr. Samuels is depriving Mrs. Barnes of any future opportunity to obtain additional psychotherapy from a disinterested professional who has no agenda aside from helping her. Should she need psychological help at some distant time, she will be forced to start from scratch with a new therapist.

As for the case of Rev. Sanderson and Mrs. Atkins, he can be credited with the awareness that he needs to get out of the dual relationship he currently has with Mrs. Atkins, whom he is counseling as well as dating. His decision to suggest that she transfer to another parish, although understandable, would be considered unethical on two grounds: First is the problematic nature of having a minister date any member of the congregation (see below). Second, Rev. Sanderson has a psychotherapeutic relationship with Mrs. Atkins that he has decided to terminate in order to be able to pursue his personal agenda of converting her into a romantic partner. Rev. Sanderson has information obtained in the context of the professional counseling relationship that he would not otherwise know about in a different setting, as well as Mrs. Atkins's long-term trust in him arising out of their counseling relationship. Terminating a professional relationship in order to pursue a personal one is considered unethical by all the major helping professionals' organizations.

A Personal Relationship Following a Brief Professional Relationship

Shortly after moving from the East Coast to a Los Angeles suburb, Geraldine, a single, 25-year-old woman, visits the emergency room of a local hospital after cutting her index finger while chopping onions. Dr. Don Ortiz, an unmarried, 30-year-old emergency room physician whom she has never seen before, sutures her finger. During the procedure, their conversation reveals that they share a number of common interests. They do not establish an ongoing doctor–patient relationship; follow-up on her injured finger is to be with her family physician. A week later she calls the emergency room, eventually is able to contact him by phone, and invites him for dinner. Is it ethical for him to accept?

Discussion

At what point in the practice of medicine does one establish a doctor–patient relationship that precludes engagement in an intimate personal relationship? Clearly, during the emergency room visit Geraldine and Don had initiated a professional–patient relationship. But was it an ongoing one? Can she be considered a former patient a week later? This case is less clear-cut than the two

previous examples. The American Medical Association's 1991 guidelines quoted above suggest that the context, length, and intensity
of the medical relationship determine whether a subsequent sexual
relationship is ethical. Many ethicists would not be overly concerned about a sexual relationship begun after an isolated minor
emergency room visit. Yet, consider another possibility: What happens if Geraldine does not regain normal use of her finger, and
subsequently learns that Don's medical treatment was negligent,
in that he failed to diagnose and repair a ruptured tendon in her
finger? How will the new personal relationship impact her ability
to evaluate her options? Would she follow a different course of
action if she were not personally involved with Don?

An Intimate Relationship with a Family Member of a Patient or Client

Dr. Susan Lowenstein, an unhappily married, 40-year-old psychiatrist, asks Tom Wingo, the married twin brother of her catatonic
hospitalized patient, Savannah, to come in to provide additional
information on his uncommunicative sister. In the course of several interviews, Tom provides much useful knowledge about the
traumatic childhood events that he and Savannah experienced,
culminating in the revelation that he was sexually molested by his
father. This admission results in the fragmentation of his macho
persona and of his history of resistance to emotional vulnerability.
These personality problems had brought his marriage to the crisis
point. As Susan and Tom enter into a sexual relationship, he begins to work through his childhood trauma and learns to express
his feelings more openly. He is eventually able to return to his wife
as a more open and caring husband.

Discussion

This fictional case will be familiar to readers of the book *The
Prince of Tides* by Pat Conroy, or viewers of the film adapted from
this novel. The justification for considering as ethical the sexual

relationship between Dr. Susan Lowenstein and Tom Wingo, the patient's brother, was that Tom was not technically Dr. Lowenstein's patient (never mind that both were married). However it might be rationalized, she was in fact engaging him in therapy, while the chemistry between them evolved from the painful and intimate revelations he uncovered. She then took advantage of his vulnerability to obtain relief from her own marital difficulties. Medical ethicists today are uniform in condemning this psychiatrist's behavior as exploitative and unprofessional.

Not uncommonly, primary care physicians, lawyers, or ministers are faced with an ethical dilemma when they become interested in pursuing a personal relationship with a pediatric patient's mother or an elderly client's daughter. Although the various professional ethical codes do not specifically address this issue, the helping professional needs to remember that romancing the relative would create a dual relationship with patient or client as well as the relative, leading to a potential conflict of interest. The practitioner contemplating such a relationship might well ask, How will my personal relationship influence my treatment decisions? Will I consciously or unconsciously be predisposed to be more involved and attentive to this case? Take more risks? Give the patient special attention? Be more or less likely to withdraw life support? Be less objective? Charge the same professional fees for care? And what would happen to my personal and professional relationships with family members if I were to mishandle the management of this case or commit a serious error?

A Personal Relationship Between a Minister and a Member of the Congregation

Rev. Steven Prince, age 30, a widower with a 2-year-old daughter, notices an attractive young woman who has recently joined his church. When he learns she is single, he asks her for a date.

Erica Walters, a single, 30-year-old statistician in a small midwestern town, joins a new church. She finds the new minister, who is also unmarried, very attractive, and she invites him to dinner with the intention of letting him know she is interested in a romantic relationship.

Discussion

It is often difficult to meet a compatible life partner, and the church or synagogue is traditionally an approved place to make social contacts. Is there a problem, then, for an unattached minister to use his congregation as a meeting place? The ethics of a dating relationship between minister and parishioner rest on the role definition of a minister. The key factor here is that the minister, in his role as "leader of the flock," is considered a potential resource for help and solace. Even if a previously unknown parishioner does not need his professional help now, she may do so in the future, but this will not be possible if they develop a sexual relationship.

Marie Fortune (1995), a minister who has written extensively on the ethics of sexual relations between clergy and parishioners, states:

> Sexual contact by pastors with parishioners is a violation of professional ethics that not only undercuts an effective pastoral relationship but, also, is exploitative and abusive. It is not the sexual contact per se that is problematic but the fact that is takes place within the professional relationship. The relationship may be formal, such as between a pastoral counselor and a client, or less formal, such as between a pastor and a parishioner currently serving on a parish committee or seeking pastoral support during a crisis. Regardless of the particulars, the relationship between a clergyperson and those whom he or she is called to serve is a professional one within which sexual activity is inappropriate. [p. 30]

Although all major religious denominations prohibit sexual relations between the minister and a parishioner if either is married, different religious denominations have different guidelines regarding sexual relations between an unmarried minister and a single parishioner. In many Christian churches, any sexual relationship outside of marriage would be regarded as sin, and would disqualify a minister to continue in his role; the issue it would raise is the sin of fornication; the question of sexual exploitation is not usually addressed. Less fundamentalist churches are forced to examine the issue of sexual exploitation in more detail.

The Code of Professional Practice of the Unitarian Universalist Minister's Association (1997, p. 13), for example, states, "If I am single, before becoming sexually involved with a person in the congregation, I will take special care to examine my commitment, motives, intentionality, and the nature of such activity and its consequences for myself, the other person, and the congregation." This vague statement does not address the fundamental leadership role of the clergyperson which gives him increased power vis-à-vis the congregation.

Marie Fortune (1989) disapproves of *any* sexual relations between a minister and a parishioner:

> Sexual contact within a professional relationship creates a dual relationship; that is, both a love relationship and a counselor/ client relationship. This dual relationship undercuts any possibility of an effective counseling relationship. Such a relationship is based on a parishioner's being able to have confidence in the knowledge and authority that the clergyperson brings as pastor or counselor and to know that this knowledge and authority will not be misused. The parishioner also must be able to trust the pastor to respond to her best interest, and not the pastor's self-interest alone. Sexual contact between the two seriously diminishes these important factors and hence, the professional relationship itself. [p. 103]

The reality, however, is that in rural communities there is often only one professional in any given category in the entire community—one physician, one minister, and so on. Should they remain single and celibate? Must they date outside their own community? Some congregations address this issue by having full-time clergy for counseling duties exclusively and others have the ministers abstain from all psychotherapy and refer parishioners to a church-based counseling center or to trusted community professionals (Lybarger 1997, personal communication).

Romantic or Sexual Relationship between Attorney and Client

Alfred North, a divorced, 45-year-old attorney handling the divorce of 40-year-old Jennifer Sawyer, finds her very attractive. Her husband filed the action after becoming involved with a young professional woman with no children who works in his company. Jennifer is distraught over the divorce, worries about how she will manage returning to school and raising her children, and welcomes Alfred's nurturing and support during the proceedings. Prior to settlement of her divorce proceedings, they begin a sexual relationship.

Robert Linder, a single, 38-year-old divorce attorney, who exclusively handles divorce cases, invites Marjorie Dawkins to dinner and a movie six months after concluding his representation of her in her divorce.

Ellen Green, a 33-year-old unmarried businesswoman, is attracted to her tax attorney and invites him for a romantic dinner.

Discussion

The legal profession has lagged behind the medical and mental health communities in considering the ethical ramifications of practitioner–client sexual relationships. Although the 1998 edition of *Model Rules of Professional Conduct* of the American Bar Association (ABA) discusses various aspects of dual relationships such as gifts, business relationships, and representing relatives, it says nothing about sexual relationships with clients. In 1992, however, the ABA's Standing Committee on Ethics and Professional Responsibility adopted a nonbinding ethical opinion that advised attorneys to avoid sexual contact with their clients:

> A sexual relationship between lawyer and client may involve unfair exploitation of the lawyer's fiduciary position, and/or significantly impair a lawyer's ability to represent the client competently. . . . All of the positive characteristics that the lawyer

is encouraged to develop so that the client will be confident
that he or she is being well served can reinforce a feeling of
dependence. . . . Moreover, the client may not feel free to
rebuff unwanted sexual advances because of fear that such a
rejection will either reduce the lawyer's ardor for the client's
cause or, worse yet, require finding a new lawyer, causing the
client to lose the time and money that has already been invested in the present representation. [Jorgenson 1995, p. 266]

The ABA committee suggested that, because of the enhanced
potential for conflict of interest, impaired judgment, and betrayal
of confidences, an existing attorney–client relationship creates a
climate in which sexual relations are rarely appropriate.

Different state bar associations have dealt with this matter differently. Under the New York State Bar Association's Code of Professional Responsibility, (1992) only matrimonial lawyers are specifically barred from having sex with their clients. However, the
code also states that all lawyers are prohibited from "accepting employment if the exercise of professional judgment on behalf of the
client will be . . . affected by the lawyer's own . . . personal interests."
This statement presumes that the attorney is capable of determining whether his personal relationship is affecting his representation, which may not necessarily be true.

The California Bar Association similarly hedges its rules. Rule
3-120 of the State Bar of California (1995) states, in part, "A member shall not continue representation of a client with whom the
member has sexual relations if such sexual relations cause the
member to perform legal services incompetently." Again, this rule
does not acknowledge that a vulnerable client might be unable to
freely choose whether or not to engage in sexual relations with the
lawyer, regardless of the efficacy of the representation; moreover,
it implicitly permits the attorney to turn over the case to another
attorney in order to continue the sexual relationship, a scenario
that is explicitly considered unethical by the professional associations of physicians, psychologists, and social workers.

The issue of sexual relations with former clients was not addressed by the ABA, but such relations may be inadvisable. For one,

we can ask, in parallel with a professional relationship between psychotherapist and client, when is the case really over? Every time there is a legal question about child custody or renegotiating the divorce settlement, the attorney is cast back in his or her professional role and will again represent the client. For another, any future relationship will be contaminated by the nature of their initial relationship, which was one of power inequity. It is likely that the client confided to her attorney many intimate facts about herself, whereas he did not reciprocate. By virtue of the prior relationship, he is unilaterally in possession of information about her that he can use for his own ends in the subsequent sexual relationship. Some people might therefore conclude that it would be unwise for them to develop a romantic relationship.

Intimate Relationship between an Adult Student and a Teacher or Professor

An unmarried, 32-year-old assistant professor asks a 19-year-old undergraduate student who is in his class to go out to dinner and a movie with him.

An unmarried, 35-year-old assistant professor asks a divorced 35-year-old undergraduate student who is in his class to go out to dinner and a movie with him.

A single, 20-year-old undergraduate student invites her major professor to a romantic dinner.

An unmarried, 35-year-old college professor asks a 30-year-old graduate student in a different department for a date.

Discussion

The area of sexual relations between faculty and students is one of active discussion and disagreement in academic circles. There is general consensus on the impropriety of the situations exemplified by the first three cases, as stated, for example, in the Code of

Academic Integrity of the University of Arizona (1997): "Consensual sexual relationships between teacher and student, where the teacher has authority over or responsibility regarding that student, are considered inappropriate and could lead to disciplinary action." The professor who wants to date a student in his class is in a position to affect her grades; his suggestion of a date is therefore clearly in the realm of sexual harassment. Even if she is the one who makes the advances, the potential for exploitation is still present, and it is the responsibility of the professor to decline her invitation. Moreover, in the present academic climate, the professor who dates a student over whom he has authority, even if the student initiates the invitation, is risking his career by opening himself up to the possibility of subsequent charges of sexual harassment.

On the other hand, a professor and a student in a different department, as in the fourth case, might be considered two adults who meet in the workplace, and if he is truly not in a position to influence her grades, then many people would consider a sexual relationship between them acceptable.

A Professional Relationship That Is Preceded by an Intimate Relationship

Judy Jones and Bob Ellsworth were college sweethearts in California. Their relationship ended when Bob traveled to the East Coast to attend medical school, and each married someone else, but they remained in contact and considered each other friends. Twelve years later, when Bob returns to California to set up practice as a plastic surgeon, Judy makes an appointment to consult him about some scars she'd like to have removed.

Discussion

Is there an ethical problem here for Bob if he has Judy as a patient? Surely not everyone needs to refrain from using the professional expertise of their friends.

GRAY AREAS IN RELATIONSHIPS OF UNEQUAL POWER

In Chapter 4 we discussed cases where there was a clear-cut power differential, so that a sexual relationship clearly constituted sexual exploitation by one party. However, as shown in this chapter, in many relationships the power differential falls on a continuum, and decisions about the appropriateness of a personal relationship between the two people must be made on a case-by-case basis. Each of the scenarios described in this chapter have one common denominator: the two people are potentially engaged in dual relationships with each other. In all but the last scenario, a preexisting professional relationship that involved varying degrees of power inequity was followed by an actual or potential intimate relationship; in the last scenario, the personal relationship came first. In deciding whether a romantic or sexual relationship is likely to be exploitative, the degree of power inequity must be examined; the greater the inequity, the greater the potential for harm and abuse.

Our two primary assumptions are (1) that it is generally harmful to the person in lesser power to have a sexual relationship with the professional, even when the former considers the relationship to be consensual; and (2) that the person with less power is not able to give truly informed consent to the relationship and is therefore vulnerable to exploitation. Not everyone agrees with these assumptions. For example, feminist scholar Daphne Patai (the sister of one of the authors) who is opposed to regulation of personal affairs, writes (personal communication, 1996):

> The discussion of power seems to me confused: on the one hand it is standard sexual harassment definitions; on the other it's the "one person has more special knowledge of the other." Does that mean secretaries shouldn't date their bosses because the secretaries quite typically know far more about the bosses' private affairs than vice versa, and could exploit them? Or do the different kinds of power differentials cancel one another out?
>
> Say a powerful, wealthy, 70-year-old man marries his immigrant housekeeper. By current standards, this is sexual ha-

rassment/exploitation (on his part, need I say). But of course, the woman could well be seen as the exploiter, using her youth and sexuality. Why should this be regulated?

If one takes seriously the issues you raise, they certainly could be applied across the board to many other comparable situations. I for one do not want to hand the state, or professional organizations, and least of all my fellow citizens with their often petty and irrational motives, the power to regulate *my* personal life because it doesn't fit into *their* categories for approved relationships.

Society used to regulate personal relations in all sorts of ways far more than it does today. Interracial relations were out; same-sex relations were out; even religious intermarriage was frowned upon. And cross-class relations were of course particularly unacceptable. Let's not go back to those days.

We have quoted this scholar at length because her views are held by many thoughtful people, and also because they contrast with the support many feminists express for a model that aims to prevent exploitation of those in positions of lesser power, who are generally women.

It is true that in many, if not in most, relationships there are factors that create a power differential; one person may have less education, less sex appeal, less money, lower status in the community, less prestigious employment, less influential friends, or a physical or psychological handicap. There also may be a significant age disparity. The aging millionaire and the young woman are one example. Or a person may be providing a service and thus has greater power; for example, your house painter may deliberately miss a few sections of your wall, or take forever to finish the job, if you offend him; your financial advisor may give you bad advice if you spurn his advances; your attorney may not pursue your case forcefully if you reject him sexually; your boss may choose not to promote you if you don't respond to his sexual offers.

Should all these relationships be regulated? Clearly not, but we believe that some of them should be, and so does the law. We reject the argument that because not all relationships should be regulated, none should be. It is certainly true that some intimate relationships that began as fiduciary relationships of unequal power never harmed either party. But in our experience, harm occurs often enough in such relationships that certain categories of such relationships should be considered ethically untenable.

An important point is that it is not personal relationships that are being regulated, it is *professional* relationships. Generally the law looks at the practice of a profession as a privilege, not a right, which the state has the obligation to regulate for the good of the public. Alabama attorney and therapist Charley Shults (personal communication, 1997) writes:

> If the woman I can't live without walks into my office today in order to see me as a therapist, I am free to decline to enter into the therapeutic relationship in order to pursue the personal relationship, and to refer the potential client to someone else. I would question my ability to function very well as a therapist in such a situation anyway.
>
> If this is a client I have been seeing for several years and if this is indeed true love that I can't live without, I am free to walk away from my practice, give up my license, and pursue the relationship that will make my dreams come true. If pursuing a personal relationship with the client is really that important, then the professional must be prepared to make whatever sacrifices are required. That is a part of the responsibility that we assume when we take our oaths, or subscribe to a code of ethics, that requires us to refrain from any personal or dual relationship with a client or patient for our own gain. The point is that regulating professions, and the professional relationship with the client or patient, is totally appropriate.

We believe that the dependency and power inequity in professional relationships fall on a continuum. The potential for harm when such relationships become sexual depends on many factors, including the type of services rendered, the expectation for future services, whether the professional relationship still exists and if not, how long since the professional relationship ended, the length of time and depth of intimacy of the professional relationship, the transference and countertransference that has developed, each individual's psychological makeup and emotional health, and the cultural background of the people involved, which can strongly influence how each person's gender role and professional status is viewed by the other. Some situations have unquestionable potential for damage, whereas others are less clear-cut. When the potential for harm in professional relationships is high, regulation by law or by a professional organization may be the most effective way to protect the consumer.

One of the most important points that we emphasize in this book is our belief that the person with lesser power is often not in a position to choose freely whether or not to engage in a sexual relationship with a person of greater power, and that the person is often unaware of this lack of freedom. This factor is often unrecognized. The parishioner who is favored by her minister may consider his romantic interest in her to be the best thing that ever happened to her; the negative consequences may become evident only at a later time. An understanding of this point is crucial to making sense of our opposition to this type of dual relationship.

MAINTAINING APPROPRIATE PROFESSIONAL BOUNDARIES

This chapter has discussed the difficulties encountered when two people find themselves in dual-role relationships. In such relationships the boundaries that normally define interactions between people are not clear. It is often not possible to avoid dual-role relationships, particularly in small towns or in subcultures where people are thrown together both socially and professionally, for example, in a university community, on a military base, within a religious fellowship, or in any minority community. Another example is a twelve-step fellowship (Alcoholics Anonymous or its many offshoots), where a physician or counselor may find himself attending the same meeting as his patient or client. Professionals might prefer to attend a different meeting, but this may not be possible if there are only one or two meetings of that fellowship in town.

In situations where multiple relationships are unavoidable, it is particularly important to be very aware of what are appropriate boundaries and to make conscious choices about the nature of the relationship. Sexual boundary violations are usually the last in a series of other boundary violations. Maintaining appropriate non-sexual boundaries in professional practice is the most effective way for the clinician to minimize his or her risk of violating sexual boundaries.

Epstein and Simon (1990) developed an educational tool they call the exploitation index, which is a series of thirty-two self-assessment questions for therapists who wish to assess their behavior and attitudes in their own practice. As Epstein and Simon readily admit, "teaching aids and self-assessment checklists are unlikely to be of much direct help for therapists possessed of the more malignant forms of denial described in the sexual exploitation literature" but might forestall sexual abuse in the "majority of individuals whose behavior and attitudes fall in the transitional or prodromal category—exploitative activity that may seriously interfere with the efficacy but that has not yet (and may never) become gross abuse" (p. 455).

From the exploitation index (pp. 455–462) it is possible to adapt a series of recommendations for helping professionals to maintain appropriate nonsexual and sexual boundaries. Guidelines for maintaining appropriate nonsexual boundaries include:

- Avoid giving patients or clients the impression that they have a special status. To this end, see clients only during office hours, do not condone chronic lateness, missed appointments, being seen routinely on a walk-in basis, or not paying bills (unless specific payment arrangements have been agreed to); avoid social contact with patients outside of clinically scheduled visits.
- Avoid excessive self-disclosure. Do not reveal personal information about yourself in order to impress the client. Avoid

discussion of your personal problems. Be sure your disclosures are for the client's benefit, not your own.

- Avoid barter, especially of personal service. It is wisest to be paid for your services only with money.
- Limit dual relationships to the unavoidable: Do not accept friends, family members, or office staff as clients. Avoid diagnosing and prescribing for them (this is often very hard to do!).
- Recognize that much of your appeal to the client is due to your professional role and to transference; do not be seduced by the client's appreciation and admiration.
- Do not ask clients to do personal favors for you.
- Don't try to influence clients to support political causes or positions in which you have a personal interest.
- Don't undertake any business deals with clients.
- Don't accept valuable gifts from clients.
- Set an appropriate interpersonal tone in the workplace: observe appropriate dress codes, and refrain from making sexual comments and innuendoes, and comments or jokes about patients.
- When dual relationships are unavoidable, be aware of the pitfalls, monitor yourself, seek consultation from trusted colleagues or a supervisor, and document carefully.

This list is intended to assist the clinician in making conscious choices about exceptions; it is not a rigid set of rules requiring strict adherence. Special patients or clients are found in every professional practice; they constitute one of the gray areas that are the focus of this chapter. Clinicians are advised to identify special clients or patients and evaluate their interactions and boundaries in these relationships to determine if the patient's special status is safe and appropriate for the practice. For example, if giving out the home telephone number to patients is not the clinician's usual practice, it may be completely appropriate to do so for the family of a patient who is dying, extremely ill, or in crisis.

Dual relationships constitute one type of boundary crossing. Boundary crossings, however, are not the same as boundary violations, and need not necessarily be avoided. The most effective way to prevent the former from becoming the latter is to be clear about the existence of a dual relationship when you are in one, and recognize the risks involved. When in doubt, consult a trusted colleague, someone who will ask the hard questions and challenge any questionable practice.

Another list of guidelines can assist the clinician in maintaining appropriate sexual boundaries:

- Avoid intrusive questions about the patient's personal or sex life. Be sure that all such questions are relevant to the patient's care and are for his/her benefit rather than your own.
- Avoid inappropriate touching. Be aware of where your body is relative to the client's. Be sure that hugs and pats are for the client's benefit, not yours. On the other hand, remember that touch in itself is often therapeutic (Hunter and Struve 1997).
- Do not make sexual comments about the client's body.
- If you are a physician, give the patient privacy to get undressed and, during the examination, explain examination techniques before you perform them. Have a chaperone in the room during examination of sexual areas.
- Have a strategy for dealing with seductive patients. This may include noting in the chart any direct or indirect romantic or sexual overture the client makes, and obtaining supervision and assistance in determining what to discuss directly with the patient and when to transfer the patient to another clinician's care.
- If you are sexually attracted to a patient or client, discuss this with a trusted colleague or a supervisor, not with the client.

Professionals exploit clients for various reasons. Among the sexually exploitative professionals assessed by Irons, 8 percent were exploitative on the basis of naïveté, in that they lacked an understanding of professional boundaries and had difficulty distinguishing professional from personal relationships; 18 percent were in life crisis and turned to the patient for nurturing to meet their emotional needs, or as part of a rescue fantasy; 54 percent were addicted to drugs and/or sex; and 23 percent had primary psychiatric illnesses including Axis I disorders, personality disorders, and psychotic illnesses.

Reviewing these checklists can assist clinicians in identifying behaviors that are potentially risky, and planning for changes in their future professional techniques. Such a strategy is useful for a minority of potentially exploitative professionals, primarily those who are naive or in a life crisis. Professionals who are addicted or suffering from a psychiatric illness are likely to be in too much denial or incapable of benefiting from procedures that require self-awareness.

Part II

Categories of
Sexually Exploitative Men

6

Archetypes of Sexually Exploitative Males: Role in Assessment and Treatment

> Thinking about sense objects
> Will attach you to sense objects
> Grow attached, you become addicted
> Deny your addiction, it turns to anger
> Become angry, you confuse your mind
> Confuse your mind, lessons of experience are forgotten
> Forget experience, you lose discrimination
>   *Bhagavad Gita* (translation modified
>   by one of the authors [R.I.])

Hundreds of millions of years ago, when the animal kingdom was beginning to differentiate into various subgroups of phyla, genera, and species, interactive diencephalic (old brain) and hypothalamic (area for basic drives and motivations) centers evolved, and have remained part of the central nervous system for most of the animal kingdom. Within these areas there developed a system that provided neurochemical rewards for behavior that was useful for survival and procreation. The final common pathway was the stimulation of areas that can roughly be termed the "pleasure centers" of the brain. Various simple compounds functioned as neurotransmitters, which brought to the pleasure centers either stimulation (reward) or motivation to avoid the behavior in the future (aversion). These neurotransmitters were able to stimulate the pleasure centers, and as a result the centers put out chemicals of their own. Various stimuli and behaviors produce different neurobiochemical pathway responses. Research in this area is just beginning to produce useful information regarding these pathways.

The results of the latest research on these phenomena resonate with the introductory quote from a spiritual/religious text that is over 2,500 years old. When a person begins to focus attention on another object, a desire complex is formed. A desire complex is a matrix of likes and dislikes, attractions and aversions, preferences and judgments within the superstructure of the personality. We respond or react to a desire complex with conditioned, patterned perceptions, and approving or disapproving judgments. These are often unconscious.

The entire world as we experience it is composed of objects we desire, those we wish to avoid, and those toward which we feel neither attraction nor aversion. Levine and Levine (1995) describe desire as a merciless restlessness of the mind that experiences itself only as dissatisfied longing for what it does not have. It is an inherent part of being human and as such is neither sinful nor evil. Yet either the gratification or frustration of desire leads us to emotional states we associate with pleasure, power, pain, and suffering.

When compulsive thought revolves around a desire complex, craving often evolves into ritualized behavior directed at gratification. This drive to appease craving can become powerfully reinforced. The Buddhists have a phrase for this. They describe such dissatisfied longing as "hungry ghosts," which come to possess us. The frustration of desire leads to anger, violence toward oneself or others, pain, loss of self control, powerlessness, and suffering. Attachment to desire leads to punishment by desire, which we refer to as addiction.

We may awaken one day to find that we are standing at a turning point. And in that moment we may recognize that our best thinking and attempts to control our lives have brought us to this critical juncture. This is a painful state, often experienced in addiction long after promises of abstinence from mood-altering substances, fidelity and dedication to a primary relationship, and avoidance of certain behavior have been broken many times.

One may have experienced many losses, tried to recover for other people, and yet the regressive pull back into addictive behavior recurs. When one is sick and tired of being sick and tired, when one wants to be free from the addictive cycles of acting "in" (getting religion, abstinence, avoiding high risk behavior, dieting, being "good") and acting out, then one may realize one is ready to mindfully investigate the series of events through which desire leads to behavior that is self-destructive and self-defeating.

Desire can dominate mind through compulsive thoughts and euphoric recall. It can also lead to an unwillingness or inability to control our impulses. The time between a thought of "I want" and an action to appease that wanting becomes so short that there is no longer the ability to consider the consequences of the action. Table 6–1 gives an overview of the process.

Table 6–1. A Cartography of Desire

When desire forms in the mind, it inspires intention.

Memory reinforces inclination.

We move toward the object of desire in an attempt to possess and/ or control it.

Our intention forms around the anticipated satisfaction and gratification.

Our mood begins to change.

We may engage in ritualized patterns that may bring pain and suffering.

We seek to secure control over the object of desire through attachment.

The intention (wanting) of an object is strongly reinforced by state-specific learning. State-specific learning is experienced when a person recognizes the ability to learn or recall certain information of images in a given mindset and perhaps in a given environmental setting. It can also be associated with certain chemically altered states of consciousness. One can see oneself reenacting scenarios from past experiences, especially when they have been powerful and meaningful. Note the voice within (intention) that urges us to act upon each wanting. Many of these desires are mundane and innocuous; yet some are so compelling that they begin to dominate personal values and priorities. The drive to reserve and protect the object of desire for our personal (and often exclusive) use is the foundation of pathological fears and narcissistic defenses.

As Levine and Levine (1995) point out so beautifully, "Intention is the weak link in the chain of events [by which desire acts itself out]. Desire seems uninvited and quite compulsive in its leanings. And note the voice which says we must act on each wanting. Although the contents of desire are quite seductive, when we are relating to desire rather than from it, its process becomes painfully evident" (pp. 154–155).

We need to appreciate that the shift of perception involved in relating *to* desire rather than *from* desire is subtle but very important. When we live from our desires, they control our actions. When we live in relationship to desire, mindful and honest with ourselves about our motives for wanting, then we are able to choose whether to act upon our desires. When a person is caught in addiction he is no longer able to relate to desire. Desire may then become all consuming as eloquently shown in this eighteenth-century poem.

A Drinking Song

Bacchus must now his power resign—
I am the only God of Wine!
It is not fit the wretch should be
In competition set with me,
Who can drink ten times more than he.
Make a new world, ye powers divine!
Stock'd with nothing else but Wine
Let Wine its only product be

Let Wine be earth, and air, and sea
And let that Wine be all for me!
—William Broome 1689–1745,
The Oxford Book of English Verse, 1940

It is not even desire that is the cause of our pain, but identification with it as our fate, our only alternative. Caught in the neurobiochemical jaws of an addiction, the addict sees only his desires, his needs, his suffering, his despair. The shift in perception to relating to desire as a human characteristic allows one to appreciate that he habitually gives in to desire, and now the pain of others, the needs of others, and the alcoholic who still suffers can be seen for what they are—other manifestations of desire in the world. At this point one has genuine freedom of choice regarding any given desire. The goal is not to abolish desire but relate to it rather than from it.

Rene Guyon (1934) said,

> To abolish the torment of desire is no doubt the most radical cure for all human ills: unfortunately it is beyond human strength. Desire will die when the appearance of desirability has become eliminated. That disease of the mind which we call desire compels us to create inaccurate ideas which do not correspond to things as they are, but as we should like them to be, ideas which are the result of an effort of imagination. In this way the element of sex can be driven out by the element of the impure or the horrible. [p. 171]

Freedom from compulsion enveloping a desire complex, and freedom from loss of impulse control associated with an object of desire or aversion require the desire and the intention to end the thoughts and actions, and the will to experience the living truth regarding how these thoughts and actions affect others and our perception of others. When we are truly enlightened, we use the desire for Truth, for God, to overcome our desire for lesser things. Investigation into the nature of desire becomes an opening into the heart and allows a new perspective on wanting and getting. This investigation can lead to compassionate service of others and deeper mercy and forgiveness of ourselves.

ARCHETYPES OF SEXUALLY EXPLOITATIVE PROFESSIONALS

When desire dominates the mind and leads to action regardless of the consequences, sexual exploitation can result. Some cases of professional sexual impropriety are at least partly attributable to character pathology, for example, narcissistic personality disorder or dependent personality disorder. On the other hand, defects of character are often part of addictive disease and are treatable. We have found that a useful way to summarize the categories of exploitative persons is through a set of archetypes. These facilitate easy recognition of sexually exploitative professionals and assist in explanations to concerned parties who are not trained or fluent in psychiatric diagnostic nomenclature. The archetypes are described in detail in Chapters 7 through 12.

ARCHETYPAL CATEGORIZATION

It has been helpful in our assessment program to categorize professionals who have abused power and position to exploit those they serve into six archetypes, each associated with a different treatment and prognosis. Although not classic Jungian archetypes, they possess some of Jung's flavor and utility. They are of considerable benefit as a therapeutic language to convey to the exploitative professional, peers, and regulatory agencies the nature of the misconduct or offense and to assist in the difficult task of determining the recurrence risk.

The Naive Prince

Early in his career, this type of professional feels the power of his new status and feels invulnerable. He is psychologically healthy but may have been poorly or incompletely trained with regard to appropriate boundaries. With one or a few patients he develops "special" relationships. Usually, these are women with challenging or difficult problems who possess a particular psychodynamic profile the professional finds provocative, intoxicating, and intriguing.

Subsequently, a blurring of appropriate professional boundaries leads to sexual misconduct or offenses. The professional recognizes he is involved with a patient in a relationship far beyond what he intended, and in retrospect realizes he exceeded ethical boundaries. In a short time, he is found out. The "naive prince" responds well to education, counseling, and monitoring. Princes may be naive but not innocent, and they must understand the responsibilities of power and the hazards of its abuse.

The Wounded Warrior

Following completion of training and professional initiation, this professional commits much effort and energy to serving his patients. He becomes engrossed in a demanding position. Social life and personal needs are secondary, as they were during training. He may be married and have children, but his personal validation and self-worth come from this professional mantle and a need to serve. Professional and social demands and internal struggles over wounds from the past lead him to become sexually or romantically involved with one or more patients, and he becomes more isolated. His exploits serve as a temporary escape but resolve nothing. He secretly carries guilt and shame and feels relieved when confronted.

The "wounded warrior" has no major psychiatric problems but may have situational depression. He may be chemically dependent and/or sexually addicted. He is usually early enough in his career and sufficiently invested in maintaining his professional status to successfully respond to therapy, and his rehabilitation potential is good.

The Self-Serving Martyr

This professional has progressed to middle or late career stages and sacrificed personal growth and family involvement to his career. He views himself as a suffering servant of others who do not appreciate that he is consumed by his professional duties. He becomes angry, resentful, and isolated. With "special" patients, he rationalizes and justifies exceptions to professional boundaries. Ritualistic grooming progresses to sexual misconduct and offense, often with a series of patients over a long time. When a confrontation occurs, he may be exhausted physically, emotionally, and intellectually, as well as being spiritually bankrupt.

"Martyrs" have significant neurotic conflicts, are often withdrawn, or dysthymic, and may have unattended physical maladies. They often abuse drugs and alcohol and may also be sexually addicted, or may have problems in other areas such as compulsive eating or gambling—all in an attempt to escape pain. Character pathology may be seen with obsessive-compulsive, narcissistic, dependent, or hysterical traits. They may meet the psychiatric criteria for mixed personality disorder. They are almost always professionally impaired when assessed, and their recovery is slow.

The False Lover

The "false lover" lives a life of intensity and continual high drama, dwelling on the loves and appetites of his body and mind, enjoying life on the edge, and the thrill of the chase for fulfillment of passion and conquest. Often demanding and perfectionistic, he may appear as the eternal youth. He becomes captivated by a series of women, each of whom appears for a while to meet his image of perfection, but eventually is found to be ordinary and mundane. He is charming, creative, energetic, idealistic, and romantic. He is frequently addicted to drugs and to sex or romance. Desire for adventure and notoriety may lead to high-risk behaviors and a dream to have it all—fortune, fame, career distinction, and a Dionysian lifestyle. Inevitably, conflicts arise in both personal and professional areas. Sexual exploitation takes place in and out of his professional practice. The unmanageability of his life is seen in a pattern of divorces, job changes, failed geographic cures, or legal problems.

"False lovers" usually present in denial and genuine crisis. They generally meet psychiatric criteria for adjustment disorder, psychosexual disorder with addictive and exploitative features, and at least one other active addictive disease. Character pathology may include obsessive-compulsive, narcissistic, adolescent, and dependent characteristics. Impulse control is a major concern.

These professionals are usually impaired when they come for assessment. They are best treated by addiction specialists. Rehabilitation requires substantial personal change and a commitment to a lifelong recovery program.

The Dark King

Driven by grandiosity and a desire to control and dominate, this professional is a man of power. Socially adept and verbally facile, he appears charming and charismatic. Using rational arguments, he convinces those he serves that he possesses special abilities.

He initially experiences professional success and notoriety. With time and resources at his disposal, he becomes more deliberate, cunning, and manipulative. Sexual exploitation becomes a right and expression of power, superiority, and dominance. Victims are carefully chosen to met his needs and sexual agenda.

He is therapy-wise, psychologically well-defended, and legally informed. Although "dark kings" are rare, they are the professional exploiters most frequently portrayed in the media. Possessing a rich and pathologic array of narcissistic, sociopathic, borderline, and schizoid personality disorders, often with superior intellectual gifts, they are the material from which books are made. They are usually not addicts, but their professional impairment is a risk to their patients and usually requires revocation of their license.

The Madman

This mentally ill professional has an erratic, unpredictable course in his personal and professional life. He may have a major depression with psychotic features, manic-depressive illness, or dissociative disorders, but is usually not chemically dependent. Following treatment for his mental disorder, he may perform well for periods of time and then again engage in sexual impropriety. Return to practice is possible with ongoing treatment and careful monitoring.

The six archetypes are based on over 200 professionals who were assessed by Irons over a several-year period. Table 6–2 lists the distribution of archetypes found among the sexually exploitative male professionals assessed. Because men constituted 96 percent of the sample, there were not enough women to categorize into female archetypes. Eventually we hope to be able to create a set of archetypes for women. Although there is likely to be a great deal of overlap between male and female archetypes, we anticipate some differences, and await a larger sample of women. Classifying exploitative professionals into the six archetypes clarifies their underlying motivations and helps in predicting their likelihood of rehabilitation. The following six chapters discuss each archetype in greater detail.

Table 6–2. Archetype Distribution

Archetype	*Percent*
Naive Prince	7.9
Wounded Warrior	22.7
Self-Serving Martyr	25.0
False Lover	19.3
Dark King	13.6
Madman	11.4

7

The Naive Prince

We could say that naïveté is a state of feeling which avoids the dark side of one's own motives or the motives of others. Naïveté discounts anger, fear, or greed, and assumes more goodness in the world than there is. The naive person often refuses confrontation or combat, and if thrown into it by circumstances, often fails to notice the moment of defeat. Naïveté is a failure in initiation.

Robert Bly (1989)

Kirk Warren, a married, 31-year-old family practitioner, entered into a multidisciplinary assessment after a married couple from his medical practice disclosed to one of his physician colleagues that Kirk had become emotionally involved with their 17-year-old daughter, also a patient. During this period of time Kirk had been establishing a busy professional practice. He was feeling stressed and depressed. He felt his wife was so dependent on him that he could not share his inner turmoil and emotions with her. Instead, he began spending time outside

the office with the patient, who seemed lonely and in need
of a friend. He asked her to come to his home to baby-sit his
two small children. Both Kirk and his wife came to know her
and feel comfortable having her care for their children in their
home. Over time, he shared more and more of his personal
life with this young woman. In the office, he gave her extensive birth control advice and did a pelvic examination. He also
helped her find a part-time job and lent her money. As the
relationship progressed to hugging and kissing, he became
frightened of where it was heading and broke it off, although
he continued giving her medical care. The girl told her
mother, who complained to Kirk's partners. At this point Kirk
agreed to come in for assessment, although neither he nor
his wife believed he had done anything wrong. He appeared
unaware that he had violated appropriate doctor–patient professional boundaries.

Kirk grew up in a rigid, disengaged family. He was the
oldest child in a family where the father was demeaning and
critical. His mother used Kirk for comfort and solace as he
became old enough to listen to her worries and concerns. He
became the family's caretaker, the family "hero," working hard
to live up to his parents' expectations. His self-esteem came
from his achievements. His self-worth was based on accomplish-
ment, and the home environment was very competitive. He
never felt he could measure up to his parents' expectations.
Kirk married his high school sweetheart and never had any
other sexual partners. His wife was naive and very dependent,
and he felt he had to maintain the appearance of strength and
control in the home.

Psychometric testing showed dependent and histrionic
personality traits in an immature individual. He demonstrated
low self-esteem outside of his professional persona, and appeared to be very needy of affirmation by others. He also
exhibited symptoms of dysthymia. Kirk had no evidence of any
addictive disorder. Nonetheless, the assessment team felt he
was acutely professionally impaired because of his distorted

thinking and lack of ability to maintain appropriate boundaries. He appeared at that time to be very vulnerable to boundary violation with other patients.

It was recommended that he temporarily withdraw from
practice to engage in intensive inpatient treatment, and subsequently receive education about boundaries, marriage counseling, and individual psychotherapy to deal with unresolved
family-of-origin issues. He did have excellent rehabilitation
potential. When he returned to work he agreed not to see
adolescent patients for a period of time. Four years later he
was seen in follow-up. He had returned to a full professional
practice, was finally able to see adolescents and children, and
had not engaged in any further boundary violations or ethical improprieties.

During a young professional's schooling, the instructors and
courses, the inspiration of masters, with their repositories of knowledge, and the mystique of those whose displays of talent rival those
of the ancient magicians provide him with all the education he can
absorb in the time allotted. He develops confidence in his ability
to memorize and recite the material required by teachers, completes the required curriculum, and completes the journey to
graduation. He earns a professional degree, and with it the belief
that he is prepared now to enter into an active career.

For those who enter a helping profession, there is an additional stage in this passage that involves a period of apprenticeship.
As a junior professional, he is required to begin his vocation of
public service under supervision. Senior professionals guide him
through trials, triumphs, and failures as the initiate experiences the
challenge of applying his acquired knowledge to life situations.
Long hours of labor, often extending into nights and weekends,
are not uncommon. Yet the young prince knows that the end of
this servitude under masters of the profession comes soon enough.
The great dream—to become a man of power, prestige, and privilege—is finally realized.

The young man is now touted as a hero by his family and
friends. Indeed, this journey has been long and arduous. The lau-

rel was earned at a significant price, but this is not the time to appraise the cost. The dream has come true through effort, talent, and perseverance. Dragons of doubt and insecurity have been slain. The hero has now arrived at the beginning of a new season in his life as an "ordained" professional.

This fresh spring of professional life is celebrated by the prince. For now, he has reached a milestone and may embark upon his life work. This very personal dream grew from the soul of the boy, and whispered to him that if he follows this path he might be of value in the world and prove his worth through service to others. Now the time to serve has come. Now, with a sense of exhilaration and exuberance, the young prince can practice his profession as he chooses, as he sees fit, in his own style.

During the passage to ordination, teachers have encouraged and rewarded steps to independence, and the ability to use this acquired knowledge and learned skills upon and for others. Possessing the latest theories, and knowing how to use the privileges and powers reserved for the profession with skill and dexterity, the prince is ready to engage the world, suffused with pride in his new status. Feeling almost invulnerable, he becomes enthralled with the opportunities that lie before him.

The naive prince of whom we speak is a young officer in the professional legion. He is embarking upon on one of his first assignments. He has been observed in the controlled and structured environment of the professional apprenticeship and found to be psychologically healthy, and able to perform professional duties without obvious difficulty or struggle. Now in a position to be trusted to offer his skills to the public more independently, he can savor the power and responsibility of his office. He feels confident of his ability to perform professionally, and is eager to face new challenges with energy and enthusiasm.

Prior to the formal completion of training or within the first five years or so of professional life, the prince may encounter a situation that appears to be one of the professional challenges for which he has been well trained. He offers to be of service and develops a relationship with the patient/client that at some point extends beyond the boundary of an appropriate professional–patient relationship. The blurring or violation of the boundary may not even be apparent to the prince initially. However, due to the seriousness of this violation or a culmination of smaller violations that result in a broader breach of acceptable boundaries, the level of discomfort or pain experienced leads the patient/client or, occasionally, the professional to disclose the matter to a third party. The boundary violation is then addressed as a professional ethical problem. The prince, wounded, often falls either into shock, outrage, or at times apoplexy.

Kirk is an example of a naïve prince. He was not aware of the gradual erosion of appropriate boundaries with his young patient that inexpediently led to emotional enmeshment over time. The boundary erosion progressed under the observation of his wife, who never considered this young woman's presence in their home and the attention Kirk gave her to be a violation of professional boundaries, nor did Kirk. This propensity for not carefully considering where a specific erosion in professional boundaries might lead is characteristic of naive princes. Often, the boundary blurring and erosion process arouses powerful emotions in the patient, the professional, or both. These emotions may not be easy to acknowledge or address, and for a professional with limited experience, may be far stronger and more confusing than he could have anticipated. Nothing in his course of study and training prepared him for this complication, this unexpected course of events. Suddenly, his professional persona is fractured by strong personal emotions. Now that he realizes that there is sexual or romantic tension in the relationship with a certain patient or client, the professional is unable or unwilling to choose a course of action that will defuse the situation effectively without harm to either person.

In retrospect it often becomes apparent that there were some areas of professional education that were incompletely absorbed or taught. And it is within the boundary violation that the naive prince exhibits his limited social experience and personal naïveté as well. Naive princes are often encouraged by their teachers and mentors to spread their professional wings and fly. They may overestimate their abilities and possibilities. They fall prey to inflation of their new persona and develop an immature narcissistic defense system that represses dependence upon peers or others who might monitor their professional activities. The dissociated experiences of weakness, limitation, dependence, and personal need may then be projected onto the opposite sex within the professional arena (Brien 1995).

> Jerry Womack, a married, 34-year-old psychiatrist, was referred for assessment following a single episode in which a female mental health assistant alleged that she had observed him sexually molesting an adult female inpatient. Jerry was seen examining the patient's abdomen and thighs in a ward examination room without a nurse present. He had then assisted this psychotic patient in getting dressed.
>
> Jerry was a conscientious physician who worked long hours and enjoyed his work. He was primarily a psychopharmacologist who had had minimal training in psychotherapy, transference issues, and boundary education. He had no personal psychotherapy experience. His version of the observed interaction with the patient was credible. He did not anticipate needing to examine the patient's abdomen until the moment of the physical examination, and was surprised when the woman took off her skirt and panties.
>
> Jerry seemed unaware of the seriousness of his situation and of potential legal problems. He was open and consistent in his interactions with the assessment staff and did not appear to use denial, rationalization, or justification in his explanations of the incident that led to his referral for assessment. Psychological testing showed no psychopathology. Jerry was seen as a responsible person who was deferential to authority. He reported a healthy childhood, a good relationship with his wife, and no evidence of any addictive disorder. His actions seemed to have been based on poor clinical judgment and inexperience rather than any sexual misconduct. He was not considered impaired, and was felt to be safe to return to practice. However, it was suggested that he obtain boundary

education, a mentor with whom to review his casework, and individual psychotherapy to help him achieve a better balance between his personal and professional life.

Many naive princes, such as Jerry, can be passive and naive. They sulk and are meek, and become insensitive to their own pain. They absorb attack, believing that this is a noble act. They are more than willing to bear the pain of others, particularly women. They form special relationships with certain selected people, using cloying interest to get closer to them. Such princes will risk and at times lose what is most precious to them because of a lack of the establishment and maintenance of boundaries. They may even believe that if they are sincere and honest about their violations, this will protect them from the consequences of their conduct. Naïveté creates a curious link to betrayal over time. Not only will a naive prince betray another, but others will be easily tempted to betray him (Bly 1990).

THE SHADOW OF THE GIFTED ADOLESCENT

The decision to become a professional has its price, which is often paid on the level of the self in the coin of less complete personal growth and limited experience and comfort in interpersonal relationships. This season in a young man's life, between 18 and 30, is an important one for maturation, refinement of characterological "rough edges," and appreciation of the importance of relationships in life. At this very time the young professional in training is usually drawn away from family and old friends, must spend more time in study and academic competition in order to succeed, and has less time for this important personal development. An exaggerated example of this phenomenon is the TV sitcom "Doogie Howser, M.D." In this program a 16-year-old emotionally and socially adolescent intellectual genius is expected to function as a first-year medical resident. Week after week he runs into situations for which he has received medical education, yet he cannot handle them easily or often effectively because he lacks the life experience to put the given adult situation into its proper context. In such matters intellect and textbook knowledge are of limited use. One feels his awkwardness and anxiety as he tries to determine the right course of action.

This loss of the opportunity for social maturation is the shadow from adolescence that can accompany a young professional into his career. In his striving to become an adult, the drive to achieve can become an obsession, a matter of vital importance. In the process of completing professional education and training, a person comes to see his culture and its views as being one, but not the only, way to perceive and experience the world. The path to establishing a professional career generally provides an advancement in material and economic status as well. Becoming a professional is for some a path to cultural and economic freedom. For others it is a strategy to overcome the shame they feel about themselves or their family. Others choose a professional career path in search of validation and personal security. Yet all of these diverse motives produce the energy and desire to delay personal gratification in order to achieve professional status.

In many professions, this path is demanding, and the personal growth that was not completed prior to beginning of training proceeds much more slowly thereafter. The young prince has always been a good student, intellectually gifted, and considered smart. He has been able to read material and produce the appropriate responses on tests better than most of his peers. Although he has been seen as bright and talented, the shadow qualities of inexperience and naïveté remain.

OVER HIS HEAD IN THE RIVER OF PASSION

The naive prince meets one or a few patients with whom he develops "special" relationships at some point early in his medical career. In many scenarios, these are women with challenging or difficult problems who have a specific psychodynamic profile the prince finds provocative, intoxicating, and intriguing. The professional problem may be particularly difficult to address, or the patient/client and problem present in a fashion that leads to a more detailed or intense interaction than customary. In one way or another, personal problems involving relationships with others or sexuality become a matter of interest or concern. Ongoing interactions between the professional and patient expose his personal vulnerabilities, hidden desires, and interests. Subsequently, a blurring or abruption of appropriate professional boundaries results in professional sexual misconduct or offense. The naive prince then may realize that he is involved with a patient in an illicit relationship that has proceeded far beyond anything that he intended or anticipated. Drugs and alcohol are not commonly major factors in this type of professional sexual exploitation.

The naive prince may already have been in a committed relationship with another for a number of years without any history of infidelity prior to a reported professional boundary violation or sexual exploitation. He will find himself unable to explain or justify his actions, and will commonly rely upon the defense that he had maintained good intentions throughout the interactions with the patient and the patient must have misunderstood his actions or gestures, or the patient initiated sexual or romantic actions suddenly and unexpectedly. Some report their encounters as "fatal attractions." The recent movie by the same name is an uncomfortable cinematic experience for many naive princes.

In relationships with others, particularly women, the naive prince is unable to maintain safe and appropriate interpersonal boundaries. He may have grown without understanding how to conduct social interactions comfortably and effectively. Perhaps there were few if any male role models, or perhaps he was not able to integrate this important developmental skill. His lack of experience and sophistication in this arena could be due to having a relatively sheltered childhood, or he may have suffered some early trauma or failure during the development of these social skills.

Many naive princes grow up with their fathers physically or emotionally absent and are subject to what Patricia Love (1990) calls the Emotional Incest Syndrome. In her book she describes three types of enmeshed parents. Some parents romanticize children of the opposite sex, trying to find the intimacy and companionship they have failed to develop with a marriage partner. Others become enmeshed with a child of the same sex, attempting to foster a relationship in which the child is their best friend. Emotional incest may also develop between a child and a critical or abusive parent, wherein the child is not only used for emotional support but also for the release of anger and frustration. In such families domestic violence, eating disorders, compulsive gambling, and substance dependency are not uncommon. Dr. Love believes that emotional incest relationships have two fundamental characteristics. The parent is using the child to satisfy needs that should be satisfied by some adult in his or her life. In addition, the parent ignores the needs of the child. Children who grow up in families with an emotionally incestuous parent may have boundary problems as adolescents and adults. They may see boundaries as always blurred or poorly defined. Sharing intimate details of their sexual life with others at work or feeling the burden of another's problems leads to emotional closeness or enmeshment and may make the person's motives for such involvement uncertain or an expression of romantic interest. When the expression of empathy or friendship toward another is interpreted as "a pass," sexual interest, or sexual harassment, the naive prince may react with confusion and disbelief. For such princes, learning to appreciate the need for interpersonal boundaries never appropriately established by their parents is an important step in recovery and healing.

Naive princes are often optimistic, idealistic, confident, and above all sincere. Their passion to engage in the work for which they have trained academically may lead them to venture into intense interpersonal relationships with blurred or uncertain boundaries. Their limited social and relational experience leaves them susceptible to entering into professional sexual misconduct. Princes often feel that if their motives for getting close to another person were not sexual, and they did not intend to commit an ethical violation, then they should not be judged harshly and be subject to severe consequences for their offense.

Professional sexual misconduct may be experienced by the naive prince as a sudden jolt of reality in which he comes to perceive the world (and himself) as far more demanding and complex than he had ever imagined. It is a painful and costly lesson on the way to achieving personal maturity.

CULTURAL DISSONANCE AND NAÏVETÉ

Some men leave their native culture and homeland to begin professional practice in another part of the world. Although they may feel comfortable with the language and social rules of their new country, they are not skilled in more subtle and less apparent aspects of that culture or in its underlying social structure and expectations. Such men may become naive princes in this new environment despite being older and more professionally experienced. Some boundary violations may be seen then as a type of cultural dissonance between the professional and the person served.

> Sanjay Panel, a 49-year-old physician, was referred for assessment in the wake of allegations of professional sexual misconduct. Several female patients had complained that he had touched them inappropriately during office examination. Dr. Panel adamantly denied these charges, insisted he had never engaged in unprofessional conduct with any patient, and denied any desire to touch these individuals sexually.
>
> Sanjay grew up in a wealthy upper-class family in India. He obtained his initial medical training in India, but at age 35, having completed additional medical training in the United States, he chose to make his home there. He set up a solo practice in a rural community, where he and his wife brought up their three children. As the only doctor in town, his practice was very full, and he tended to spend very little time with each patient.
>
> Psychological interviews and testing showed a defensive and guarded individual who had compulsive personality traits and some dysthymia, but indicated no evidence of a psychosexual disorder. Sanjay was somewhat unsophisticated and naive in interpersonal relationships. In his physical examinations, he was very goal-directed in his efforts to diagnose physi-

cal problems, and he tended to ignore his patients' emotions. His practice style did not include explanations for particular examination procedures, and he seemed not to understand that his actions might be interpreted by patients as sexual. In a practice examination on a member of the assessment team, Sanjay allowed contact between his pelvic area and the patient's body, but the contact appeared inadvertent, and Sanjay seemed genuinely surprised when this was pointed out to him.

The assessment team's opinion was that Sanjay was uninformed, insensitive, and perhaps unaware of how his touch might at times be interpreted as sexual by female patients, but that he did not have a sexual agenda in his actions. He was determined to be unimpaired in his ability to practice medicine, but only with several conditions: He was to have a female chaperone present for all interactions with female patients; he was to attend educational courses in appropriate boundaries in personal life and professional practice, in the signs and symptoms of sexual abuse, in distinctions between therapeutic and nontherapeutic touch, and in professional ethical boundaries; and he was to consider moving into a group practice with peer professionals.

Some naive princes may have been poorly or incompletely trained. In the process of training as a professional, their ethical foundation never fully developed. They come to recognize that they had only partially formed professional boundaries. In retrospect, they are capable of coming to the realization that they had violated ethical standards, and failed to integrate and appreciate ethical precepts. It is the ability to gain genuine insight and true integration of this important principle for the first time that distinguishes the naive prince from the other archetypes. The naive prince will have circumscribed areas of vulnerability that can be addressed and rectified, rather than an innate inability to develop or unwillingness to maintain an ethical foundation. Naïveté and passivity are both related to emotional numbness. The naive prince is asleep to the greed, ill motives, and the dark side of himself and others; in contrast, passivity is a state in which one is asleep to the responsibilities and implications of personal disclosure, love, emotional expression, and professional duty. In both situations the man will experience emotional numbness with constricted emotional expression and the frozen inability to resist engagement in seduction. The distinction between naïveté and passivity as the precipitating cause is of particular significance, for the approach to treatment and base etiology is very different.

A FAILURE IN PROFESSIONAL INITIATION

Naive princes have not been completely trained and educated professionally. We consider this deficit a failure in professional initiation. These men have not incorporated some basic precepts in the area of healthy and appropriate professional boundaries. Rather than descending into a vortex of dialogue about the reasons this can occur during the education and training of professionals, let us at least make some general comments. The educational and training process for professionals has become far more didactic and cognitive over the past five decades. In most of the classic helping professions, such as ministry, medicine, and law, for most of their existence there was for aspiring students completing their formal or textbook education a period of apprenticeship, in which a bond developed between mentor/artist/professional and the apprentice/craftsman/initiate. Ethics and boundaries were absorbed and integrated in the course of this relationship. An example of this was the training of Zhivago in *Doctor Zhivago*, by Boris Pasternak.

Essentially, the process of initiation removes the ego from the center of the universe. When a society abandons initiation and rituals, individual egos lose an appropriate means of learning this valuable lesson. Life circumstances will urge the same lesson upon the ego eventually, but perhaps in a very painful, inopportune manner. But by far the most serious consequence of not honoring the essence of the initiation process is the loss of a generational social forum for considering and appraising the nature of maturity (Moore and Gillette 1992b). This is certainly true for most of the helping professions. The process of gradually assuming professional duties in relationship with one or more older and more experienced professional superiors has been considered vestigial and has largely fallen away. Most young professionals are released as fledglings into the world to proceed far more independently and with less of this apprenticeship experience than in other eras of professional training. And one of the greatest losses in this evolution is the integration and appreciation of the subtleties and variations of the professional–patient relationship.

TREATMENT IMPLICATIONS

Most naive princes have the ability to form a solid ethical foundation, and can learn from experience. We have defined one of the crucial characteristics of this category as a failure in initiation. Therefore, education and a completion of training in areas where there are deficiencies is very effective in addressing the primary causes for boundary violation. Naive princes have been given power and position that was too potent for them to handle, and like the sorcerer's apprentice, their use of power resulted in unskillful action. If the prince recognizes that he violated professional boundaries, is not yet completely trained and educated professionally, and exhibits genuine remorse, his prognosis for recovery and professional rehabilitation is excellent. Such professionals respond well to education, counseling, and monitoring. Development of authentic maturity requires introspection and the self-directed choice to bear the mantle of responsibility for what we say and do. Those confronted at this stage are fortunate, for most avoid progressing to other archetypal categories. They often express gratitude to those who had made the effort to confront them before they progressed into a ritualized pattern.

A NECESSARY LOSS OF INNOCENCE

Princes may be naive but they are not innocent. Ethics are not to be gained merely by leaving behind or dismissing our capacity to abuse power and position, and to respond to the power of seduction. Such an ethos would be little more than self-righteous pride and hubris. To admit frankly the capacity within each of us to engage in such behavior allows us to break through our pseudo-innocence. With appreciation of this dialectic, we have become more sensitive to the genuine ethos of profession and power. We learn, often when we move closest to the dark side of ourselves, the burden and responsibility of power and the hazards of its abuse. We become responsible not only for the direct effect of our actions, but also for being as mindful as possible of the more subtle and less direct effects our actions have upon ourselves and others.

8

The Wounded Warrior

I am not a mechanism, an assembly of various sections.
And it is not because the mechanism is working wrongly,
  that I am ill.
I am ill because of wounds to the soul, to the deep emotional
  self
and the wounds to the soul take a long, long time, only time
  can help
and patience, and a certain difficult repentance
long difficult repentance, realization of life's mistake, and
  the freeing oneself
from the endless repetition of the mistake
which mankind at large has chosen to sanctify.

> D. H. Lawrence
> (Ravagli and Weekly, 1964, p. 78)

Michael Prosky, a 45-year-old clinical psychologist, was referred by his professional licensing board because a complaint had been received that alleged he had had a sexual affair with Laura, a former patient. Michael admitted to initiating a sexual relationship with the patient only two weeks after their psychotherapeutic relationship had been terminated. He rationalized his departure from ethical conduct with an elaborate explanation of mitigating circumstances. Michael indicated that this was a time of great stress for him. His wife had increased her professional commitments and was very busy, he had recently increased his alcohol consumption, and had been drinking too much the night he called Laura and asked if they could see each other outside of the terminated doctor–patient relationship as "friends." He continued the clandestine sexual and romantic affair for several months, until guilt overcame him and he ended his involvement with Laura. At that point, Michael decided to turn his life around. He disclosed the sexual affair to his wife, stopped drinking, and became involved in A.A.

Laura spent a year attempting to reignite the relationship. When she was unsuccessful, she then disclosed the past involvement to her current psychologist, and was supported in her decision to submit a complaint to the licensure board. An intensive investigation by the licensure board failed to reveal any other professional improprieties. No further complaints were brought forward against him, even after a public disclosure of his acknowledged professional sexual misconduct. Michael was regarded by his peers as an exceptionally talented practitioner. His professional practice group and hospital encouraged him to get help for his problems and offered hope that he could return to his previous professional practice.

Michael was the oldest of four children. Born with a congenital heart defect, he was in and out of the hospital and underwent several operations over several years until the problem was fully corrected. He described his father as being a problem drinker who was emotionally abusive. His mother was warm and caring, but she was frightened of his father. The task of everyone in the family was to please Dad. Michael, in particular, experienced pressure to succeed and to be the perfect son.

Extremely bright, Michael excelled in college and chose a career as a psychologist, where he could work with people and be of service. In graduate school he met his future wife, a warm, nurturing woman who seemed finally to fulfill his longing to be cared for. Their relationship always continued to be very important to him.

On psychological evaluation, he had no prominent characterological pathology on psychological testing, although interviews suggested some dependent traits. He was noted to be a well-functioning, responsible person, who had had a serious lapse of judgment associated with a time of severe stress, exacerbated by his active alcoholism at the time. The assessment team believed that Michael's diagnoses were an adjustment reaction with disturbance of mood and conduct, and alcohol dependency. The felt that as long as he addressed his sexual misconduct successfully in primary treatment, psychoeducation, and continuing psychotherapy, he would not be a danger to patients and could resume practice in his profession safely under a recovery contract, whose recommendations included intensive treatment for sexual misconduct and alcoholism, continued psychotherapy for codependency issues, and that, for the time being, he not engage in psychotherapy of women in any professional setting.

Following successful completion of treatment for these problems, he was supported in professional reentry. He continued in his individual psychotherapy weekly over the next eighteen months. During five years of monitored reentry, no further episodes of professional impropriety occurred. Michael and his wife report that their marriage is very rewarding and they are very involved in raising their two children.

When a young man completes the rites of passage into his chosen profession, he ventures forth in the world to make his mark. He has completed his academic training and period of apprenticeship. He possesses the intellectual knowledge from his curriculum of study, as well as the guidance and support of mentors and scholars. He has been told he has potential, and has received inspiration from the learned warriors and professional heroes that he desires to emulate. These are not storybook figures from fairy tales; they are flesh-and-blood giants who stride through the corridors of power and strength, wisdom and action in the course of service in his professional fortress of learning.

He has dreamed and labored for this opportunity to discover just how talented he is, how adept at applying the scientific and intellectual acumen he has absorbed in his years of study and apprenticeship, to begin the joy of professional creativity and service. Now he has been given the mantle of power and the seal of approval through ritual ceremony and public licensure or confirmation. He goes forth as a professional warrior to serve humankind.

The warrior moves forward in his early years of practice to establish himself as a professional who can help others. He begins to earn recognition, appreciation, and praise for his efforts. He gains confidence in his abilities as he experiences success in professional endeavors He is rewarded for his service to others with increased power, community stature, and material comfort. He has become a success, a hero to his family and many others.

THE WOUND

Within this warrior there is a wound. It has been there for a long time. Years of professional education, apprenticeship, and now professional practice have transpired, and the effort of achievement has facilitated the ability to keep the wound hidden. This metaphorical wound often has its inception during childhood development, before professional training was even contemplated. These wounds develop in a part of us that becomes inherently vulnerable in the process of childhood, as described in Chapter 2.

In many a warrior, the wounds of childhood and adolescence are repressed as the goals of attaining a medical, psychological, or religious education and professional training are pursued. If these wounds are not repressed, they are recalled with cognitive distortion. The events associated with the wound and any subsequent recrudescence are commonly not interpreted as traumatic or hurtful, but as a developmental stage that has been overcome and laid to rest. The warrior does not know that he carries the wound within. Or he may be aware of a nagging residual ache from an old complaint sustained in growing up. Either way, the warrior does not perceive the wound as either active or of any current importance or relevance.

Some years pass. The professional has begun to feel comfortable and confident in practice. He may find himself committing most of his time and energy to serving his patients or clients and advancing his career. This venture into the world has engrossed him in a demanding position. He feels needed and vital to his organization. Social life and personal needs are secondary to the professional roles and duties, as they were during training. He may be married and have children, but his personal validation and self-worth come from these professional activities and this insatiable need to serve and achieve. However, this level of dedication and intensity has a price. The warrior eventually begins to experience existential conflict, as repressed wounds from his past emerge and take new forms. These unresolved wounds reemerge in ways that surprise and baffle the professional.

Michael Prosky, whose case began this chapter, was congenitally wounded and sustained obvious physical stigmata as a result of his corrective surgeries, making his wounds visible to all as he progressed through childhood. He entered early adulthood with memories of his operations and of his progressive adaptation and physical recovery. They provided him with the interest and compassion for those who suffered that led him to the study of psychotherapy. He was able to address and work through his own childhood trauma as he proceeded into a career that would allow him to serve others. By the age of 45, Michael had achieved much in life and could see himself as a pillar of his community, a good father and husband. The family lived comfortably in a wonderful home and the children had every opportunity for growth and development that could be provided. Yet Michael felt that something was missing. He could not put his finger on the exact problem, but he did know he was restless, irritable, and somewhat unsatisfied in his personal and professional life.

At the time he presented for assessment he did not think he was looking for Laura, but that she sought him out and actively seduced him. Yet in the power and desire that was kindled as they came to know each other, he began to recognize his own sense of incompleteness, his hunger for a certain comfort, and his need to feel idealized and admired physically and sexually. The emotions kindled in the process reminded him of his early childhood when he was doted on and protected by his parents from overextending himself and from exposure to infections or high-risk situations, his search for validation as an adolescent, and the lost love of his teen years, with whom he discovered the pleasures of sexual intercourse for the first time. This young woman had left him a few months after their sexual relationship began for one of the high school football stars. Michael had mourned the loss of this relationship for many years, and always felt that if he had not been born flawed but rather had been endowed with athletic prowess, she would not have abandoned him. Somehow Laura reminded him of this young woman, and of the love he had always wanted. Michael had two childhood wounds of the heart, one congenital and one emotional, that accompanied him into his adult life. One was obvious to him and others, and the other lay harbored deep inside and unrecognized despite his professional training as a psychotherapist and his own past experience with therapy.

Professional demands, social obligations, and repressed internal struggles led Michael to become involved with his patient in a slow progression of steps. At first he found himself thinking of Laura after professional office visits. He took particular interest in her problems, family, and personal history. Over time he discovered that she, too, was yearning for change in her life, feeling very dissatisfied and frustrated. While treating her for anxiety and depression he made the less than fully conscious human error of believing he could also rescue her from her struggles and liberate himself at the same time. The wounds of childhood and adolescence were now being played out through regression into sexual acting out and mutual romantic projection.

As Michael became more isolated, guilty, and troubled by his behavior, as he realized that he had committed an ethical violation, he tried to convince himself that he loved Laura, just as he was convinced that his first love of adolescence was "true love." In contrast to others who have recollections of their first adolescent or early adult sexual experiences, Michael had been deeply wounded by the subsequent rejection and felt betrayed, yet at the same time inadequate as a man and responsible for the loss. The trauma was significant for him. In fact, he was able to acknowledge that he had never unconditionally given himself emotionally in any subsequent relationship. He hesitated to trust any woman completely, even his wife, fearing that she would discover his masculine shortcomings or would betray his love and commitment to another. Repressed internally, he carried the core belief that if he were to leave himself vulnerable again, he would again be hurt deeply.

Michael carried not only the physical scars of multiple cardiac surgeries but this large emotional scar. He remained fearful of intimacy and deep communication with others, particularly women with whom he was sexually involved. Laura was an idealized object of desire because she offered to nurture and comfort him, to devote her life to him, as he imagined he had been treated by his mother or could have been loved by his adolescent sweetheart.

Michael tried to hide this contemporary manifestation of his wound by keeping his relationship with Laura secret. When Laura wanted to pursue the relationship to a commitment, Michael realized he could not reciprocate. By the time the sexual misconduct was reported to the licensure board, he was ready to accept help and wanted to work for personal healing, even if he could not achieve professional rehabilitation.

George Dixon, married, a 50-year-old physician in general practice, was referred by his state's medical licensing board for assessment in the aftermath of allegations of sexual misconduct by two patients who reported that they had been inappropri-

ately examined by him. George came to admit that he had
engaged in intrusive overextensive examination of two patients
he had known and served for many years, within a six-month
period of time, a period when he said he was experiencing
major stresses at work. Full investigation concluded that these
had been isolated events in his life; there were no other prior
victims or other ethical violations.

George grew up in a strict, traditional religious family, with
a weak, emotionally absent father and a powerful, controlling
mother. The close, smothering relationship she had with her
son can best be described as emotional incest. George's job
throughout his childhood was to serve as a substitute husband
and fulfill his mother's emotional needs. George chronically
suppressed his anger and became the family "hero," gaining
acceptance through being the good son, the successful son.
Even as an adult he continued to seek her advice.

A dedicated and caring doctor, George had throughout his
successful career sacrificed his personal needs to serve others.
He was a workaholic who spent long hours in the office and
was available to his patients 24 hours a day, seven days a week.
His identification as a physician was the only source of self-
esteem for him. He considered his marriage good and his wife
supportive, but he was not really aware of her dissatisfaction
with his total involvement with his practice.

Psychological evaluation suggested that George was a lonely,
emotionally immature man who was still very attached to his
mother and had never grieved her death. He had strong dependency needs, using sex to get his need for nurturance met.
He had a strong desire to merge with another person in order to feel whole. On the outside he appeared self-confident
and authoritative, but within he felt very insecure. There was
no history of addiction or abuse of alcohol or any other drugs,
and nothing in his sexual history to suggest paraphilia or a
sexual disorder.

Initially George had difficulty understanding the harm he
had caused his patients by his sexual involvement with them,

but eventually came to recognize this as a professional sexual offense. His diagnosis included dysthymia, and, on Axis II, dependent personality traits (codependency). He was considered professionally impaired. Treatment recommendations included initial inpatient treatment for the sexual misconduct. George was advised not to return to primary care medical practice, in particular not to perform physical examinations of female patients. Part of George's current income had been coming from reviewing insurance records, and he was advised to consider switching to this work full-time.

George was a wounded warrior. Years of service had left him isolated and lonely. His sudden departure from adherence to exemplary ethical professional standards shocked many of his peers, the community, and especially his family. George met the two women in rapid succession who somehow rekindled images of the emotional bond he had felt with his mother as a young man when he served as her confidant and "little man" for a number of years while his father, a successful salesman, was physically and emotionally absent from their lives. The sexual misconduct began about nine months after the death of his mother, and during a time when his professional practice was beginning to provide decreasing financial rewards and personal satisfaction. His work had served as his primary source of validation, and he felt that his family could not understand the conflict he carried inside. His exploits served as a temporary escape but resolved nothing. He secretly carried profound guilt and shame and felt relieved when confronted by the state physician health program.

THE SHADOW OF THE WOUND

Consciousness becomes less responsive to environmental stimuli. One experiences mental dullness and torpor, as well as a general sense of personal "stuckness" or stagnation. A person may be emotionally unreactive or unresponsive as well, and an arrest in emotional development is common. Some writers refer to this as a loss of activity in the emotional body. Many men have no role model

for this activation in their personal or professional life. Moore and
Gillette (1992b) state that two marks of the uninitiated male are
wife beating at one extreme and an impotent softness on the other.
A woman who notices that a man's emotions are not activated will
sometimes offer to activate it for him. It may be that sex deepens
the integration of the physical and the emotional in women, but
this does not work for men. In passivity, without activation of the
emotions, men may live through years of relationship with a woman
without expressing anger, become secretly resentful, and feel dimly
perceived rage and passive hostility. The passive man will allow the
woman to do the expressing, the pursuing, the initiating, the
doing; his emotional expression and will to resist seduction is frozen.

A significant number of helping professionals (in our experience, over 40 percent) present for assessment sincerely believing
that they are in love with the person from their professional practice with whom they have become sexually involved. Glen Gabbard
(1995) has heuristically referred to such individuals as lovesick
therapists. The narcissistic themes often seen involve an intense and
at times desperate need for affirmation and validation by those they
serve, an insatiable desire to be loved and idealized, and a tendency
to use those served to bolster and maintain self-esteem. Others may
have borderline personality themes that leave them open to quickly
forming passionate identification with patients or clients, acting
upon these feelings impulsively, then breaking off the involvement
abruptly. Others act out of neurotic conflicts or existential frustra-
tions.

Gabbard points out that many lovesick therapists will insist that
the relationship they have with their special patient transcends any
consideration of transference and countertransference. Yet outside
this particular folie à deux the therapist's reality testing appears to
be intact. Gabbard outlines a variety of psychodynamic themes
among the lovesick that bear reiteration:

- Unconscious reenactment of incestuous longings (on the
  part of one or both parties)

- Misperceiving a patient's wish for nurturance as a sexual overture
- Interlocking enactments of rescue fantasies
- Patient viewed as an idealized version of the self (narcissistic projection)
- Confusion of professional's needs with patient's needs (an occupational hazard for therapists is to inadvertently or unconsciously gratify their own needs while they are meeting the patient's needs)
- Fantasy that love in and of itself is curative
- Repression of rage at patient's persistent thwarting of therapy
- Professional's anger at the organization or system
- Manic defense against mourning and grief
- Insecurity regarding masculine identity
- Conflicts around sexual preference (in same-sex dyads)

These themes of lovesickness, which we are calling wounds, are as operative in other types of professional sexual exploitation as they are in the therapist–patient scenarios described by Gabbard.

Patrick Stefani, a 34-year-old physician, was referred by a state medical board for a multidisciplinary evaluation after he was discovered to have engaged in a sexual relationship with a current patient. The patient, Susan, having learned that Patrick's wife had just left town, called him, indicated her interest in a sexual involvement, and invited him to come to her home. Patrick was intrigued enough to assent, but within a month the magnitude of the marital and ethical violation led him to try to break off the relationship. Susan threatened to report him to his medical board, and then began following him around, leaving notes on his car, and accosting him in the hospital parking lot. Eventually he became frightened enough to turn to his state's physician advocacy committee for help.

Patrick was raised in a rigid disengaged family with a strong ethnic and Catholic heritage, yet within which no one spoke of their feelings. There was never any physical or sexual abuse, and voices were not raised in anger. Keeping up appearances was a quality that was highly valued. Patrick's father, a practicing physician who was known as an alcoholic and womanizer, was self-absorbed and distant. His mother, frightened of men in general and of her husband in particular, considered Patrick her "special" child, her confidant to whom she turned for comfort and company. He tried to please his father by being macho and successful, and his mother by being the perfect son. Patrick grew up with a legacy of low self-worth, which was only partially alleviated by academic and professional success. At the age of 4 he received a stuffed dog as a gift. He continued to treasure this animal, sleeping with it every night. Several years later, the family dog attacked the little bedtime friend, tearing it to pieces. Patrick was inconsolable until it was repaired. He continued to sleep with this companion until about 14 years of age. He retained the stuffed animal in his possession as an adult, packed away in a box in his house.

Patrick's assessment did not yield any evidence of chemical dependency or an addictive sexual disorder. Although he had had two prior brief affairs during his marriage, neither of which involved a patient, these were not felt to be part of an addictive sexual disorder. Psychological evaluation showed the presence of dysthymia and, on Axis II, narcissistic and dependent personality traits. Because of his personal vulnerability and unmet dependency needs, he was considered to be potentially impaired and was urged to voluntarily withdraw from medical practice until his personal problems were addressed.

Recommendations included intensive treatment for his dependent personality traits and family-of-origin issues, attending a continuing education course on professional–patient boundaries, and, after return to practice, the presence of a chaperone for all physical examinations of patients. It was felt he would also benefit from long-term insight-oriented therapy.

Patrick did return to his medical practice, under a consent order with his state medical board. He followed to the letter the practice restrictions included in his recovery contract and consent order. He continued to remain in annual contact with the director of his initial assessment and has now completed more than seven years without any further boundary violations. After five years, the medical board gave him an unrestricted license. In the course of psychotherapy, he and his therapist ceremoniously retired the stuffed dog of his childhood.

Patrick was a wounded puppy. He grew up as sensitive, intense man who was very emotional and hated expressions of aggression and violence. He was caring, idealistic, passionate, and religious. He became a superb clinician who was loved by patients and colleagues alike. However, there was within him a certain sadness, which could be seen in his eyes. It would remind one of the emotion seen in the eyes of Omar Sharif in the film of *Doctor Zhivago*. This legacy of unresolved pain was visible to some of those who knew him, particularly certain women.

Patrick was determined to become a professional, and kept most people at an emotional distance during his education and training, with the exception of the woman who was to become his wife and the mother of his two children. Within him remained a deep need to be comforted and nurtured. The two women with whom he had brief extramarital affairs and the patient whom he engaged in professional sexual misconduct were for him women who offered to comfort him and assuage his pain. Their desires and drives fit together like pieces in a puzzle: his hunger to be comforted through affection and the feminine propensity to comfort and nurture. With psychotherapy, Patrick came to understand how his "wounded puppy" had become a romantic projection that brought him into conflict with his values and ethical standards. His Jungian therapist was of particular help to him in seeing aspects of his repressed feminine in his mother complex and in projected aspects of his anima. Patrick's concrete externalization of his woundedness in his stuffed animal that was carried by him into

adult life is a vivid example of the power of childhood and adolescent wounds and trauma to manifest themselves again in adult
life.

The warrior, in one fashion or another, feels emasculated by his
wound(s). This sense of impotence is often experienced as shame,
and an inner fear that his achieved status as a professional (a warrior) is not fully earned or legitimate. The wounds are often
brought to consciousness after the warrior has waged a successful
campaign to earn professional status and establish his place in a
professional group or work setting.

As Wakefield states (in Ross and Roy 1995): "Those who as-
pired to heal others were often deeply vulnerable themselves:
members of the healing professions are at risk for becoming impaired, and trying to heal the wounded can be emotionally drain-
ing" (p. 83).

The myth of Aesculapius, the "wounded healer," is an archetypal pattern in which the healer (helper) encounters or "takes on"
the illness or malady of the patient (hurting one). The healer possesses deeper knowledge of the malady, in part because of his
personal experience of being wounded in life, and from the process of "taking on" the wounds of others. Wakefield goes on to say,
"We have many names for these experiences, e.g., regression,
countertransference, projective identification, participation mystique. If the [professional's] wounds are still too raw, too unconscious, the [professional] may try to use the patient to soothe themselves (sic) in ways that are destructive" (p. 84).

The self-destructive and self-defeating ways in which this drama
may be acted out fill the pages of this book as case studies. In the
lives of so many professionals, substance abuse and dependency,
professional sexual exploitation, dysthymia and depression, and
other internal and external avenues of escape are ritualized personal portraits of struggles the professional has encountered in the
process of "taking on" these wounds of humanity in the false belief that the helper/healer has no need or right to access from
others the very services he provides as a professional. This occupational hazard is manifest in both the outward and the invisible

internal wounds of the professional warrior. Wounds of this nature are like those carried by the Fisher King from the medieval tale that is contingent to the Arthurian legends. The Fisher King found that his wounds were incurable by ordinary medical or natural means. Healing required spiritual transformation. In the recent movie *The Fisher King*, the king was facing self-induced destruction until Parcival, known as the "wise fool," intervened.

CLINICAL IMPLICATIONS

Wounded warriors are a heterogeneous group of men who at some level are struggling with one or more fundamental developmental issues. Although men in the other archetypal categories may also have these wounds, this category is reserved for those men who do not exhibit advanced characterologic or primary mental disorder psychopathology. If a man in this category has problems with impulse control or an addictive disorder, the symptoms are mild and consequences resulting from such behavior are limited. Addictive disease, including early- or middle-stage chemical dependency admixed with signs and symptoms of an addictive sexual disorder, may be found.

Wounded warriors, then, are basically psychologically healthy with limited neurotic conflicts but may have situational depression or dysthymia. Confrontation regarding professional abuse of power usually occurs early enough in their careers for professionals to have significant motivation to work toward rehabilitation. This investment to retain professional status can be used to encourage them to engage in therapy and treatment. Intensive day hospital or residential treatment with peer professionals is often quite helpful and cost-effective in accelerating the healing process and assuring sufficient engagement in the healing process to reduce the risk to public safety of professional reentry.

Often, the greatest challenge in the intervention, assessment, and subsequent treatment of men in this category is identifying the nature and extent of the "woundedness" that led to "lovesickness" and ethical violation through abuse of power and position. Re-

pressed wounds are difficult for such men to name. Once named,
it is even more difficult to fully identify the depth and nature of
these wounds, their origins in early childhood and/or adolescence,
and subtle manifestations in adult life prior to the occurrence of
a crisis in one's personal and professional life. The challenge for
any wounded warrior is to fully accept the need to heal these
wounds and integrate this part into the self. There is commonly a
strong propensity to name the wound(s), then proceed with work
on professional rehabilitation and early professional reentry if permitted, rather than doing the deeper and more fully healing personal work necessary for completion of integration and adult individuation.

PROGNOSIS

"Warriors" usually respond favorably to intervention and confrontation and at times with a palpable sense of relief that now these
personal problems can be addressed. They are motivated to complete assessment, primary treatment, and boundary education, and
are usually willing to participate in group, couple, and individual
therapy as recommended. They tend to be very compliant and
earnestly strive to develop compassion for those they have harmed.
As they come to appreciate the significance of their own wounds,
they are progressively able to have genuine empathy for those they
have themselves wounded. Professional rehabilitation potential is
good. Professional reentry is possible if such "warriors" remain in
an official state-licensed professional recovery program under a
contract that includes provisions for defined limits and boundaries,
psychotherapy, and monitoring of recovery (Irons 1991). If men
in this category are willing to apply themselves to healing these
wounds from the past, then the prospect of the wounds being reactivated in the future through behavioral acting out in personal
or professional life is very small.

As John Welwood (1996) says, we need to access the warrior
within who can help us to make use of suffering to cultivate our
capacities for strength, vision, love, faith, or humor to free ourselves
from resentment or depression.

We forge the vessel of the soul and when the heart breaks open, it marks the beginning of a real love affair with the world. It is a broken-hearted love affair, rather than the conventional kind based on hope and expectation. Only in this fearless love that can respond to life's pain as well as its beauty can we be of help to ourselves or anyone else in this difficult age. The broken-hearted warrior is an essential archetype for our time. [p. 237]

9

The Self-Serving Martyr

Shame, guilt, pride, fear, hate, envy, need, and greed are the inevitable by-products of ego-building. They call forth the polarity of inferiority feeling and power drive. They are the shadow aspects of the first emancipation of the ego.

Edward C. Whitmont
(in Zweig and Abrams 1991, p. 46)

Gerry Welters, a married, 50-year-old optometrist, was court-ordered to the assessment program after he was convicted of frotteurism, having fondled a series of patients, primarily teenage girls, during the course of examinations to fit them properly for glasses or contact lenses. An outraged teenaged girl left his office and immediately disclosed his conduct to her mother. They proceeded directly to the local police station and filed charges of assault against him. When the charge hit the local paper and nightly news, several other patients came forward with complaints that were presented to the state professional licensing board. Two of these victims also filed criminal charges against him. He was arrested, and, after posting bond, released. In response to an arraignment, he agreed to complete an assessment of his physical and mental health.

Gerry recalls that in childhood he was fondled several times by an adult neighbor. He told his parents, but they simply advised him to avoid the neighbor. His father was rageful and demanding, and in fact dictated Gerry's choice of career. The boy attempted to assuage his father's anger by being the perfect son. An extremely bright student, he did well in school and followed his father's direction in career choice. Outgoing and friendly, Gerry developed a large circle of friends. As a young adult, he managed his stress through gratifying himself with drink, sports, and sexual activity with women.

Gerry married young and considered his marriage to be solid and his wife supportive. Shortly after beginning his optometry practice, he began to touch patients inappropriately whenever the opportunity presented itself and the risk of being confronted was very low. This practice continued, and in fact escalated in frequency and intensity over many years. During his assessment he also admitted to having fondled young women who came to his home to baby-sit his children. He recalled well over a hundred occasions of taking indecent liberties in and out of his professional practice over a period of more than twenty years.

His psychological testing showed Gerry to have strong narcissistic elements, with a great deal of underlying anger that at times was strongly expressed as rage and then quickly dissipated. He characterized himself as perfectionistic, but at the same time saw himself, in projective tests, as a cute little boy. Underlying his narcissistic image was a low self-esteem, profound shame, and deep insecurity. In interviews with the director of the assessment program, he revealed that he utilized sexual acting out to escape from feelings of frustration, anger, and inadequacy. Over time he developed tolerance to the level of inappropriate touching necessary to produce excitement and relief; he began to take increasing risks.

Several years prior to his assessment, Gerry had been diagnosed with anxiety disorder. His use of tranquilizers did not deter the progression of his addictive and compulsive sexual perversion.

Gerry's primary diagnosis from his assessment team was paraphilia (frotteurism) and generalized anxiety disorder. In addition, on Axis II, he had pronounced narcissistic personality features. Professional impairment was clearly present. It was recommended that he withdraw from his optometry practice and enter inpatient treatment for his paraphilia.

Gerry had been thinking of leaving his practice permanently, and decided it would be easier for him to avoid further sexual acting out if he were not in professional practice. He successfully completed his inpatient treatment knowing that he would be unable to obtain support for return to professional practice. With vocational counseling he was able to make a decision to change careers. He committed to ongoing psychotherapy and attendance at a twelve-step program for sexually addicted sex offenders. Five years later, he was seen again and reported that he was continuing to pursue personal recovery. He was involved in a new field of work, one in which he did not have direct physical contact with others. He engaged in a prolonged legal battle with his disability insurance carrier for more than three years before an appeals court awarded him disability payments from his professional disability policy.

Young men's voyage out in the world to make their mark becomes a personal odyssey filled with struggles and campaigns. Noble allies and treacherous foes serve as protagonists and antagonists, urging them into battle over causes that seem to have importance. Wars are waged, territory gained and lost, battles fought, and honors bestowed on the heroes. Much has been seen and felt, and the scars of battle may seem to have accumulated more than honors or personal gains for the veterans. For those who have pursued a professional path, the journey has taken them from education, to professional entry, and on to the establishment of a professional career over a span of ten to fifteen years. The professional has defined an area of expertise and proficiency. By now he has attracted advocates as well as detractors, who are vocal in the community expressing their opinions. And, like the officer returning home from a life of ongoing campaigns, his family has adjusted to his career and may not always take note of the ways that his ongoing crusade to help others has worn away at his vitality and idealism. Career success has provided significant benefits and privileges, but not without extracting a price. For the martyr, work has become his life, his raison d'être, his primary if not sole source of validation and affirmation. The martyr defines himself by what he does and whom he serves, and judges himself by assuming the results are derived from his service contributions. He has heard his virtues extolled by many a grateful recipient of his time and service, yet praise and thanks never seem to be enough. He still feels as if his efforts are never fully understood or appreciated.

A warrior becomes a martyr gradually over time; there is seldom a clear dividing line. Years of fighting for others take their toll on the warrior, and he becomes more weary, burned out, and jaded, less connected to his ideals and altruism. More motivated by attrition than altruism, he becomes increasingly defensive and rigid in his professional philosophy and practice.

Many men learn the code and subtle power derived from martyrdom in their families of origin, and often from their mothers. The role of the suffering servant is adapted through masculinization and professionalization, with the expectation that a certain deference has been earned through the sacrifices made for others. The martyr arises in the professional as years of service create a certain comfort with power and expectation of privilege. This expectation evolves into a belief that certain powers and positions have been earned and are now inalienable rights to which the professional is hereafter entitled. The martyr comes to believe his competence and expertise are state of the art and should not be questioned, espe-

cially by the lay public. He would be amused if what he knows to
be professional confidence would be inaccurately referred to as
arrogance. He comes to ramble through the halls of his professional arena with ease and a defined professional image and de-
meanor, sculpted over the decades.

Yet the martyr is wearing a mask. Underneath this professional
persona, he is angry and troubled, a private man with a growing
list of gnawing resentments. Having repressed his innate
woundedness for years, he finds himself stuck in a formidable
existential bind. He arrives at a somewhat jaded view of himself as
a suffering servant of others who cannot and do not fully appreciate his dedication and the sacrifice he has made on their behalf.
He feels consumed and burdened by his professional duties to the
point of personal depletion and emptiness. He has relegated so
much of himself to his professional duty that he has nothing left
to offer his friends, family, or himself. He is worn out by weari-
ness before he can even begin to enjoy or appreciate his personal
and family life after work. His professional persona is worn so much
that he cannot easily determine if he is being what other people
want him to be or displaying his authentic self.

Over time the martyr forms a mental lament, which encapsulates his resentment and rage. Consciously or unconsciously, verbally or nonverbally, he begins to intone a personal incantation that
encapsulates his struggle and his desire for liberation. It may run
something like this: "I have done so much for so many for so long
that this time I deserve this indulgence, this minor gratification,
for I serve an uncaring, unappreciative public." The martyr makes
rationalized and justified exceptions to professional boundaries with
"special" patients or clients, characterized by emotional enmeshment and a blurring of roles he plays in their lives. When a confrontation with abuse of power cannot be avoided, the self-serving
martyr may mount a formidable defense. Denial, rationalization,
minimization, and intellectualization are common defenses used
against allegations of boundary violations and professional misconduct. However, as the archetypal pattern progresses and increased
depression, despair, and consequences of unethical conduct and

abuse of power set in, martyrs become emotionally and intellectually destitute, as well as spiritually bankrupt.

Gerry Welters had a number of characteristics we attribute to self-serving martyrs. He had labored intensively to become a successful professional, and had become a well-known figure in his hometown. He was active in community events, generous in providing services to the poor and disadvantaged, and very involved in his synagogue. He was a skillful entrepreneur as well, and had accumulated a great deal of material comfort and financial security over the years. However, he had always been a restless, driven man who had great difficulty stopping to enjoy the fruits of his labor and good fortune.

At the time of his assessment, Gerry had to admit that he could not remember exactly when or where he began to enjoy "accidental" contact with women as his arms would brush along the sides of their breasts while he completed their examinations. Over time, it became a kind of game, a contest that offered sensual excitement and mental diversion from his long hours and repetitious refraction measurements in his office. He never considered his actions harmful or traumatic to his victims. At first, he believed that the legal proceedings and public disclosure were a form of personal harassment fostered by envy and misunderstanding. He could not imagine why people would think of him as a pervert or sex offender, for he would have never considered getting sexually involved with any of these young women. He resented the media for creating a scandal merely to sell newspapers and increase their market share of viewers. He was convinced that he was the victim here, unfairly and unjustly singled out for punishment.

Gerry struggled in primary treatment, and found that he progressed much more slowly than most other patients. He persisted in seeing himself as different from others who were receiving treatment for professional sexual misconduct or sexual offenses committed outside of professional practice. He bristled when he was accused of suffering from "terminal uniqueness." He became increasingly agitated and angry in treatment as consequences from his behavior continued to accumulate and create additional pain and losses in his life and for his family. For Gerry, personal recovery was a slow and painful process.

Terence Rhymer, a married, 50-year-old Protestant clergyman, was referred by church authorities when, under a certain amount of duress, he disclosed a history of extramarital affairs over many years that had progressed to involvement with several female parishioners over the preceding five years. Each of the women was at a vulnerable stage in her life, experiencing some personal crisis, and he was in a position to provide pastoral counseling with the emotional support she needed at the time.

Father Terence was surprised and dismayed that he was dismissed from his job when he had voluntarily disclosed the facts to his superior. He was resentful of the church's lack of emotional support of him and felt that its actions were unfair. He did not seem to recognize the damage he had caused the women with whom he had been sexually involved.

Terence grew up in an alcoholic family. Having an emotionally unavailable and physically abusive father, Terence took on the responsibility of providing emotional support for his mother and younger siblings. Becoming a minister seems to have been his strategy for dealing with his shame and low self-esteem. All three children eventually became alcoholics, although Terence was able to stop binge drinking some years back and to maintain a controlled drinking pattern.

Psychological evaluation showed that Terence was very proud of his ability to help others, which was very important to him. His self-esteem hinged on his helping others, as well as on validation from women. Testing showed him to have much alienation and anger, as well as significant dysthymia.

The assessment team diagnosed Terence with a sexual disorder with addictive and exploitative features, as well as with alcoholism in remission. In addition he was found to have narcissistic, histrionic, and dependent personality traits. The team agreed with the church that Terence was professionally impaired; they recommended inpatient treatment for sex addiction, to be followed possibly by a day program at a chemical dependency treatment center. He was advised to abstain from alcohol. Upon return home he agreed to continue with individual psychotherapy and attendance at twelve-step programs. The assessment team approved of his plan to take on a teaching job, and to consider reinstatement into the ministry at some future date.

Self-serving martyrs often exhibit a pattern of professional sexual misconduct that is unique to the individual, and continues over an extended period of time. Generally, there is a series of variations on this characteristic theme. A defined pattern of grooming progresses to boundary violation and sexual misconduct and offense, often with a series of patients over significant lengths of time. The patterns of ritualization can carry symbolic meaning associated with many of the steps, or can represent a repetition compulsion played out over and over. The martyr tends to act out sexually primarily, if not exclusively, within the professional arena. His victims tend to display a general, if not specific, profile of physical and emotional characteristics. These characteristic patterns are important to elucidate, for they are necessary to successfully treat professionals in this category.

The martyr may see his psyche fractured, split by these secret relationships into a part that has masochistic or sadistic features. The masochist is often trying hard to be a "nice guy" while internally harboring passion, aggression, and rage. The masochist often has features of a dependent personality, and loses a sense of his authentic self as he labors to be what he believes other want him to be. His sense of value is based on professional performance and how others view him. He struggles desperately to be accepted, to be liked. The unconscious fear is that others could never like him if they really knew him for who he is.

Moore and Gillette (1992b) write:

> The masochist is naive in proportion to the "thickness" of his repression barrier. He is the cheerful guy who tries to befriend everyone, who looks for the bright side of everything, and who

glibly recommends ineffectual philosophies. [He] cannot deal with the forces of [seduction/evil] in his life. Fearful of acknowledging his own rage and sadism, he cannot face the reality of the rage and sadism in others. He is often the armchair philosopher, or a pacifist. The masochist is largely private. He is quiet and patient with others even when they are aggressive toward him. In many other ways he allows himself to be victimized. He will do so because he feels he cannot afford to release his pent-up demands for self expression. If he were to do so, his aggressive self-expression might burst forth in an explosion of rage. He is afraid of what his hostility might mean about him and his attempt to masquerade as a saint. [p. 127]

Dr. Glen Gabbard, psychoanalyst at the Menninger Clinic, considers masochistic surrender a primary category in his typology of sexually exploitative professionals (Gabbard and Lester 1995). These helping professionals permit themselves to be progressively tormented by persons they serve and eventually exploit. Gabbard describes a typical scenario of a male therapist who feels badgered into increasingly escalating boundary violations. The patient, often a victim of past sexual exploitation, may demand some concrete demonstration of love such that the therapist extends hours, holds the patient during sessions, and accepts entreaties for more intimate contact. Pleas escalate to demands for sexual involvement that the therapist feels compelled to oblige.

These therapists characteristically have problems dealing with their own aggression. As the patient's demands escalate, the therapist's resentment and hatred of the patient grows. "The patient may accuse the professional of not caring. The ensuing guilt feelings lead the professional to accede to the patient's demands so that aggression in either member of the dyad is kept at bay" (Gabbard 1995, pp. 142–143).

ADDICTION

In contrast to masochistic surrender, abandonment to the intoxication of seduction can lead to a very different behavioral pattern, that of addiction. Addiction serves to soothe the masochist and his

aggression, precipitates regression emotionally, and provides a disinhibition that promotes sexual acting out. This becomes an ex-
cuse or justification for departure from professional ethics in the
course of sensory gratification using a patient as the object, and
the abuse of power as a means to an end. The masochist completes
the transformation to sadist. In this respect the self-serving martyr
fulfills the definition of addiction which Henri Nouwen describes
in his book, *The Return of the Prodigal Son* (1992):

> Our addictions make us cling to what the world proclaims as
> the keys to self-fulfillment: accumulation of wealth and power;
> attainment of status and admiration; lavish consumption of
> food and drink; and sexual gratification without distinguish-
> ing between lust and love. These addictions create expectations
> that cannot but fail to satisfy our deepest needs.
>
> As long as we live within the world's delusions, our ad-
> dictions condemn us to futile quests in the "distant country,"
> leaving us to face an endless series of disillusionments while
> our sense of self remains unfulfilled. I am the prodigal son
> every time I search for unconditional love where it cannot be
> found. [p. 43]

An alternative dynamic often seen is that of chronic depression, in which the wounded warrior turned self-serving martyr over
a period of years enters the "dark forest" or, as St. John of the Cross
describes it, the "dark night of the soul," and seeks some escape
or solace through the use of mood-altering substances and/or
sexual acting out. The obedient and dutiful life turns burdensome.
Outwardly, the professional was faultless, much like the elder son
in the parable of the prodigal son from the biblical gospel of Luke.
Yet there is so much resentment among the "just" and the "good,"
so much condemnation, judgment, and prejudice. Nouwen describes such an elder son this way:

> It is in the spoken or unspoken complaint that one has never
> received what was due that the elder son can be heard. It is
> the complaint expressed in countless subtle and not-so-subtle
> ways, forming a bedrock of human resentment. Undue sensi-
> tivity to little rejections, little impolitenesses, little negligences.

That murmuring, whining, grumbling, lamenting, and griping that go on even against will and reason. Condemnation and self-condemnation, self-righteousness and self-rejection keep reinforcing each other in an ever more vicious way. When seduced by it, it spins me down in an endless spiral of self-rejection. . . . Complaints lead to what is most feared: further rejection. [pp. 72–73]

Self-pity and shame serve to increase the level of dysthymia and despair, and reinforce the conviction that one is deserving of punishment and damnation. In such situations professional sexual misconduct and offense come to represent a professional suicide attempt. With treatment, many of these martyrs come to see themselves as "suffering servants" if they are harmed again in the course of service to others. In time, some may integrate their suffering, and understand and come to terms with their abuse of power.

CLINICAL IMPLICATIONS

Self-serving martyrs commonly present for assessment or treatment in crisis from the consequences of abuse of power and position. Their pattern of exploitation extends over time, and may include repetitive, ritualized patterns of thought and action. The professional may have attempted a series of geographic cures when the consequences of his behavior would be looming, or he presents as a fixture of his community who is suddenly exposed as a threat to public safety. He may present as physically and emotionally drained and clinically depressed. He may have unattended physical maladies.

Addictive disease is common, often in a pattern of controlled chemical use associated with covert unmanageability, mixed with sexual addiction, compulsive eating, or gambling—all in an attempt to escape pain. Significant neurotic conflicts, if present, commonly revolve around narcissistic injury or fear of financial, legal, and social consequences. Characterological pathology may be seen, with obsessive-compulsive, narcissistic, dependent, hysterical features, or mixed personality disorder.

PROGNOSIS

Martyrs are almost always professionally impaired by the time they arrive for assessment. Withdrawal from practice and inpatient treatment are usually required. Recovery often progresses slowly, and further primary treatment in an extended care facility dedicated to professional patients may be helpful. Civil litigation and marital discord are common, and disciplinary action by the licensing board is almost certain. If the professional commits himself to recovery and successfully completes primary treatment, his prognosis and rehabilitation is fair but varies from case to case.

Shame is one of the dominant painful experiences of the self-serving martyr. Suffused with grandiose fantasies of professional importance and indispensability, unmodified by realistic, empathetic, caring interactions, these men face a repeating series of disappointments and failures in which they never achieve their ambitions or perceived true potential. They feel empty and worthless behind their professional mask, because their inner world harbors so few sustaining objects, ideals, and experiences. Their shame is experienced as they fail to realize these grandiose ambitions and do not attain anticipated honor and entitlement, aspects of their narcissistic defense against a threatening and uncertain world (Morrison 1986). The failure to establish and maintain close, meaningful, and satisfying interpersonal relationships contributes to the sense of persecution and isolation.

The shame over this inner and outer emptiness and repeated disappointments is accompanied by depression. Too often the depression is pharmacologically treated, but the underlying despair and concomitant shame that lead to it are not addressed.

There are martyrs who cannot attain even a modicum of genuine self-acceptance, who cannot believe that anyone could possibly accept them as they really are, and who see the failure to maintain their own lofty idealistic standards as proof that they are inadequate and inauthentic. This lack of self-acceptance and acceptance from others is a central existential dilemma that needs to be a primary focus of treatment.

Professional reentry is often delayed and subsequently restricted. Generally eighteen to twenty-four months are required to complete the treatment and recovery necessary to allow professional reentry, even in the cases with more favorable prognosis. Career transition may be desired or necessary because of the financial and emotional demands and length of treatment, ongoing therapy, and rehabilitation.

Many martyrs struggle in their personal relationships as well. Dedication to restoration of trust and credibility with family and marital partners is a challenging task. Many marriages do not survive the demands of early recovery. Many spouses are unable to recognize their own need for therapy and recovery from dysfunctional marital roles that evolved over many years. With concerted effort and sustained support, marriages can improve, and couples can bring intimacy and new meaning into their lives and their marriages.

10

The False Lover

Robert Drake, a 51-year-old family practitioner, came to evaluation because his wife threatened to leave the marriage unless he stopped drinking and having extramarital affairs. Over the course of his marriage he had had perhaps fifty sexual partners, generally in the context of a protracted romantic affairs. Most of the women he was involved with were either mothers of his young patients or nurses and other hospital staff.

Bob did not feel that his sexual behavior had compromised him professionally or personally. "Anything between consenting adults is okay as long as it doesn't hurt anyone," he said. He believed that the affairs had been fun for both him and his partners, and that no one had gotten hurt. He attributed his affairs to his wife's lack of interest in sex, and did not believe he had experienced any adverse consequences of his behavior other than causing his wife pain.

Bob considered himself a shy man, uncomfortable in social situations, but sensitive and caring. He had no friendships aside from the women he was romancing. His only in-

terests were work (which he described as "fun") and reading—
and until recently, drinking alcohol. He had drunk heavily for
many years, experiencing severe consequences such as blackouts and one arrest for driving while intoxicated (DWI), and
he had given medical care after hours while intoxicated, but
he believed that his drinking had not affected the quality of
his work. At his wife's request, he had quit drinking about a
year before coming to evaluation. In retrospect, he recognized
he was drinking as a way to medicate painful feelings and to
escape problems.

In childhood, Bob was a well-behaved, compliant only
child who never gave his parents any trouble. His father was
an alcoholic who had multiple affairs, and a very inconsistent
parenting style. Bob's mother was very controlling, and he
related to her by being the perfect son. The family "hero," his
external accomplishments provided honor for him and his
family and proved that his mother and father were successful
parents.

Bob enjoyed living life intensely, and tried to squeeze
every drop of pleasure out of his life. A major stated goal was
to have fun, both with women and in his job. At every hint of
pain or other negative emotion, he would escape into either
planning or carrying out some "fun" activity. Bob enjoyed interacting with the stream of female patients who came into
his office, and he enjoyed a long series of romances. Bob's
secret life was a source of both pride and shame for him.
Dedicated to avoiding pain, he prevented himself from reflect-
ing on what was missing in his life by regularly drinking himself to sleep while at home.

Despite experiencing two powerful addictions for many
years—alcohol and sex—Bob suffered relatively few consequences. He was still in his first marriage, had had only the
one run-in with the law resulting from driving while intoxicated, and had managed to avoid both detection and any serious errors when rendering medical care while intoxicated.
As a result, he was very much in denial about the severity of

his problems. He was unaware of potential legal consequences of engaging in sexual relationships with the mothers of his patients, including possible loss of his license to practice medicine. His alcoholism was currently inactive but untreated, so that he was at high risk for resumption of drinking. He considered his main problem to be his wife's intolerance of his drinking and multiple affairs.

Bob's evaluation found that in addition to his two addictive disorders, he had narcissistic and dependent personality traits. He was not professionally impaired, although at risk. He was referred to inpatient treatment for sexual addiction and chemical dependency, and could return to practice afterward.

Each person is endowed with a unique array of gifts and talents. At crucial points along the life journey, decisions must be made as to how one invests these resources, along with one's time, health, and energy. Graduation from an academic undergraduate or graduate program does not guarantee that one will honor the ethical commitments of a profession. The false lover might consider such traditions somewhat pedantic and maudlin, outmoded and unrealistic. He wants to enjoy the benefits of his profession: power, prestige, and privilege.

Professional life is savored by the false lover not as a mantle that was ordained, but rather as a commodity that one paid for and earned, one he can use as he sees fit. False lovers often view their profession as a job, a necessary labor that provides a means to support a comfortable life, rather than a healing ministry or an altruistic end in and of itself. If one must work, then it makes sense to the lover to get the greatest reward he can for his efforts. In meeting the requirements to be a professional, he is now able to command some well-paying position.

The false lover often appears as Dionysian figure who has never fully matured. He seeks out the most intense experience and gratifies every possible desire. In reaching adulthood and attaining professional success, a man may carry forward his desire to live a life of intensity and continual high drama. This need appears to have greatest pleasure if it can be accomplished while maintaining

career and social respectability. The false lover dwells on the loves
and appetites of his body and mind, enjoying life on the edge, and
the thrill of the chase, for fulfillment of passion and conquest.
Often demanding and perfectionist, he may appear as a *puer
aeternus* (Von Franz 1981), remaining an adolescent too long.

> Many a contemporary hero typifies what Jung referred to as
> the man dominated by the *puer aeternus,* the archetype of the
> eternal son. This archetype is typical of male adolescence,
> where its appearance is developmentally normal, but when
> carried into adult life represents a failure to grow up psycho-
> logically. The *puer* is largely a product of the mother-complex;
> he seems unable to assume responsibility for his own life and
> fails to make a serious emotional commitment in relationship.
> The *puer* must always have an escape hatch—another relation-
> ship, another project, or another move—as a way of avoiding
> the business of settling down in life. He is described as living
> a provisional life as well as one of false individualism. The *puer*
> often lives dangerously. His arrested development is attributed
> to a failure of initiation, to take the natural steps toward ma-
> turity. The exaggerated masculinity encountered illustrates one
> pole of the *puer.* The other is equally exaggerated in the fe-
> male direction, resulting in a darling boy quality, still too closely
> identified with the mother. [Pedersen 1991, p. 102]

The false lover becomes captivated by a series of women, usually in and out of professional life and practice, each of whom appears for a while to meet his image of perfection. But each is soon
found to be ordinary and mundane. His preoccupation dissipates,
and he moves on to project his ideals and desires on the next
woman, hoping she might satisfy his every need. He is charming,
creative, energetic, idealistic, and romantic.

Robert Drake is a vivid example of the *puer aeternus* who has
been able to use his youthful charm for most of his adult life to
hedonistically pursue his own gratification and self-aggrandizement.
For him, the pursuit of perfection and romantic ideals was focused
on sexual involvement with women. They, however, served as objects to be used, without consideration of their needs, feelings, or

interests. In Dionysian fashion, he used alcohol to distort his memory of traumatic events, and to assuage his guilt and shame. The pursuit of women—the "chase"—was actually envisioned as a romantic search for the ideal woman, a narcissistic projection of his own anima.

> The anima's projected image appears to be at a developmental level that corresponds to an inner development of feminine qualities. For this reason, a man is going to be unconsciously attracted to women with a developmental level similar to his own. The particular images of the anima, which are present at any given period of a man's life, span the spectrum of all female personifications. Each image represents a particular developmental achievement in a man's early identifications with the feminine. These images include the adolescent men who tend to be flighty, unstable, and unpredictable in their relationships. They may move from one relationship to another. They are often superficially charming and can have a lofty romanticism that can be flattering and seductive. They are frequently infatuated, but their enamored attachments are short-lived. Rather than being neglected by their mothers, they more frequently have been overindulged and consequently have an inflated sense of self. Their pride is easily injured, and they feel unrecognized and undervalued. If this type of anima-possessed man ever does settle down, they can become a warrior—a compulsive achiever and little sense of realistic limits in the outer world. [Pedersen 1991, p. 37]

Henry Joliet, a married, 38-year-old internist, was referred for evaluation by his medical board following complaints of sexual impropriety with patients. Henry had met a series of women with whom he became sexually involved. With his encouragement, a number of them subsequently became his patients. Because he considered himself a caring person, he felt that by becoming their doctor he would assure them good medical care. He considered these women to be "special" patients— he would undercharge them, make special efforts to see them in the office on short notice, and would even make house calls when they had medical problems.

To Henry, the intoxication of seduction was even more powerful than the actual sexual relations. He was enthralled by the intensity and intrigue, involving clandestine phone calls and assignations, romantic candlelight dinners at secluded restaurants, and complex encounters out of town. He had been involved with only one woman at a time, felt a great romantic bond with each one, and continued to regard them as friends and as nice people after the sexual relationship ended. His wife did not know about these affairs, and he was very concerned to maintain secrecy so as not to hurt her.

Henry's sexual relationship with his first wife began with great passion and frequency, but after the first child was born she lost her sexual interest. She was no longer willing to engage in new types of sexual activity, and Henry found himself very bored sexually; the romance was gone. Except in this arena, they were compatible, and for several years he met his sexual needs through fantasy with masturbation and pornography. At work he was exposed to many attractive young women—hospital employees, pharmaceutical representatives, nursing home staff, and family members of his patients—and eventually began a series of romantic affairs. He blamed his wife for forcing him to pursue other women. Nonetheless, he felt very responsible for her comfort and welfare, so he made sure she did not know of the affairs. In retrospect, he recognized that additional motives for maintaining secrecy were to avoid conflict, shame, and public disapproval, and not to risk losing his family.

When he met Julie, however, he felt it was "true love." Julie was a young, very attractive nurse. Having been sexually abused in childhood by her stepfather, she had grown up to believe that sex is the most important sign of love. She also believed that intensity was the prime manifestation of intimacy. Her beliefs closely fit Henry's needs. She thrived on the intrigue and secrecy, and she gave highest priority to pleasing Henry sexually.

Having found his perfect woman, Henry divorced his wife

and married Julie, overcoming his guilt feelings. Within a year, however, he began to find her less exciting and his marriage confining, and soon thereafter he became involved with another woman. This pattern continued right up to the time that a female patient, having learned she was but one in a long series of lovers and therefore not as "special" as she had previously thought, reported Henry to his state board of medical examiners. This report, followed by the coming forward of several other former patients with whom he had been sexual, was the crisis that brought Henry to assessment.

Henry considered his childhood to be stable, and his mother loving. His father was rigid and distant emotionally. Henry was a good student. He had never abused drugs, nor was he involved in any other addictive behaviors.

Henry's assessment revealed hidden anger and frustration against women. At the same time, he felt a need to take care of them and he tended to romanticize relationships. Henry did not recognize the boundary violations involved in having the same person as both patient and lover; he thought the only ethical problem with his affairs was that he was married at the time. The Minnesota Multiphasic Personality Inventory (MMPI-II) showed dependent and narcissistic personality traits. The MacAndrews subscale of this test, which measures addiction potential, showed a high value for impulsivity.

Henry was considered to be professionally impaired because of his addictive sexual disorder, and he was advised to withdraw from medical practice. It was recommended that he enter inpatient and then residential treatment for sexual addiction, and in addition obtain education on appropriate practice boundaries and on victimization and exploitation of patients by health care professionals. He was thought to have good rehabilitation potential after treatment, although it was likely he would need careful monitoring and a structured practice environment.

Henry represents another type of false lover, the *puer* who idealistically pursues each engaging relationship with a woman to its natural conclusion. As his own limitations in relationship and expression of intimacy within a committed relationship become evident, he experiences further pain and suffering. In the search for relief, for the woman, the goddess, he again casts his projective eye outward to find yet another prospect who may provide him with the attention and affection he desires.

Von Franz (1981) sees the *puer* as a man in search of his mother goddess. Each time he is intrigued by a woman, he later discovers that she is a mere mortal. Having experienced her sexually, "the whole fascination vanishes and he turns away disappointed, only to project the image anew onto one woman after another. He eternally longs for the maternal woman who will enfold him in her arms and satisfy his every need. This is often accompanied by the romantic attitude of the adolescent" (p. 2).

> Charles Sorenson, a married, 45-year-old physician, was referred by a state impaired-physicians' program because of sexual advances to a female patient. She had filed a complaint that Charles had kissed and fondled her in the office. He had previously had other complaints filed against him, and had promised himself to stop the behavior, but his pattern of fondling patients continued. In addition to the patient who complained about him, he had had multiple affairs, occasionally with patients, but more frequently with nurses, other hospital personnel, or women he met socially. His first affair with a patient occurred while he was in medical school. Charles believed that the patients wanted more than just a professional relationship with him and had always been flirtatious. He attributed his own behavior to his wife's lack of interest in sex, and reported that his affairs were a way of getting additional attention and affection that he didn't get from his marriage.
>
> Charles's mother was an alcoholic; his father was rigid and easily angered. Charles responded by becoming very compliant and an excellent student. Fearing his father's rage, he suppressed his own anger. At age 10, he was molested by a male teenage neighbor who assured Charles that he was just edu-

cating him about "what boys do." The abuse continued for several months and became a secret that Charles kept to himself right up to the time of his assessment. As he grew older, it became very important to him to prove to himself that he was thoroughly heterosexual.

In college, Charles began to drink heavily, a pattern that continued for many years. His colleagues noted that he drank while on call. At times he experienced blackouts. At one point he was able to decrease his alcohol consumption, but noted that his sexual activity then increased.

In assessment, Charles was noted to be immature and to want to please. He demonstrated much guilt and shame over his behaviors and appeared sincerely motivated to change. In addition to his dual addictions, he was diagnosed with dependent personality traits. He was considered currently impaired professionally, and was referred initially for inpatient treatment for his alcoholism, with plans for subsequent treatment for sexual addiction. His professional rehabilitation potential was considered very good.

Treatment was a challenging experience for Charles. He struggled with the disease concept of addiction, and required extended treatment in a residential program to appreciate the link between his alcohol dependency and his addictive sexual disorder. He needed to overcome anger, resentment, and resistance to the need for prolonged treatment. Treatment was first directed at personal recovery. Marital discord and conflicts, and legal problems resulting from professional sexual misconduct were continuing distractions. After several months, Charles was able to begin the second phase of treatment and could start to address issues that could lead to professional rehabilitation.

Following successful completion of primary treatment, and a period of outpatient therapy and intensive participation in twelve-step programs in his home community, Charles was given an opportunity to return to a supervised, limited practice about eighteen months after the initial intervention. Since then he has been able to return to a full-time medical practice. He and his wife have reconciled their differences, and are active in twelve-step programs. Charles and his wife are also active in Recovering Couples Anonymous.

Each of these case examples depicts common themes that are typical of the false lover. For these men, status and community approval was important. They belonged to the right social group, owned the right cars, lived in the right neighborhood, and went to the most glamorous vacation spots. They paid attention to their clothes and grooming and liked to be seen with important people.

False lovers are adolescents, seeking to remain eternally young. Indulging in activities that may enhance their youthful appearance, such as health clubs, tanning salons, and hair transplants, appeals to them; so does romance with a younger woman. False lovers try to live life to the fullest, to maximize the choices and opportunities that come their way. Intrigue, romance, and high drama provide excitement. Compartmentalizing their primary relationship from their romantic and sexual affairs results in a secret life, which may be experienced as living a sort of Jekyll and Hyde existence. Strong dependency needs combine with a strong drive to engage in the roles of caregiver and rescuer. The false lover's risky behaviors guarantee powerful feelings of guilt, shame, excitement, and of living life with intensity and high drama.

Gluttony, which is the fulfillment of needs to excess, is played out primarily in the sensory arena. False lovers are often sexual both in and out of professional practice. Easily bored, they are more attracted by the thrill of the chase and conquest than by an ongoing sexual relationship. The sexual behaviors of the three persons described fit the criteria of addictive sexual disorders. Each man demonstrated loss of control over the sexual behavior, continuation despite adverse consequences, and preoccupation or obsession with the activity. Potential consequences included loss of career and of marriage, public humiliation, lawsuits, and danger to health from irate husbands or sexually transmitted diseases.

False lovers do not understand the concept of balance and

moderation. Rather, their propensity to live to excess brings the belief that "if some is good, more is better." Gluttony is also expressed with other concurrent addictions, particularly alcohol and drugs. Bob's drinking was simultaneous with his sexual acting out. Charles, in contrast, tended to use his addictive behaviors alternately rather than simultaneously. He became aware that his sexual acting out escalated when his drinking decreased. Workaholism was also a common theme, and one of the men had episodic problems with compulsive eating. Living life to the fullest, fulfilling all one's desires, was a goal for all the men. They saw themselves as nice, caring, concerned, hard-working professionals who were entitled to have life's good things.

Another common feature was denial and distorted thinking. All the men blamed their wives for the affairs, and Bob formulated his primary problem as being his wife's unwillingness to let him pursue his chosen lifestyle. He did not think anyone was hurt, and believed that sex with adults was okay under any circumstances so long as it was consensual. Neither Bob nor Henry recognized that sex with patients was unethical, and only Charles, who had already been threatened with the loss of his license, recognized that such behavior had potentially devastating consequences for his career; nonetheless, Charles had continued the behavior, believing magically that there would be no consequences.

On the personal level, there was denial of the harm done to the spouse and to the marital relationship. The diversion of attention to the drama and intrigue of extramarital romance intensified the lack of intimacy in the marriage. Sex was dull compared to the affair, and the mundane concerns of the household contrasted vividly with the excitement of illicit romance. Life was lived on two levels, and the false lover became an accomplished deceiver.

Love may become the expression for signs and symptoms of addiction, as described by Carnes (1991). Desire for adventure and notoriety may lead to high-risk behavior and a dream to have it all—fortune, fame, career distinction, and a Dionysian lifestyle. Inevitably, conflicts arise in personal and professional life. Chemical dependency in the middle or late stage is frequent. Sexual exploitation takes place in and out of professional practice. Loss of control and unmanageability are often seen in a pattern of divorces, job changes, failed geographic cures, accidents, and legal problems. False lovers generally meet the criteria for adjustment disorder, psychosexual disorder with addictive and exploitative features, and at least one other active addictive disease. Characterological pathology may include obsessive-compulsive, narcissistic, adolescent, and dependent characteristics. These can represent a primary diagnosis, complicating treatment of other diagnosed disorders. Impulse control is a major concern.

TREATMENT IMPLICATIONS

False lovers usually present in significant denial and genuine crisis. Trusting in the adolescent myth of invulnerability, they can concoct and play out outrageous and complex life patterns that will not easily be reconciled or resolved. The nature of their problems generally extends into personal, family, and professional life. Someone could be simultaneously facing bankruptcy, professional licensure investigation, civil litigation, divorce proceedings, and DWI charges. The accumulated stress and consequences can promote either a hypomanic or a depressive response. Hypomanic responses involve elaborate and, at times, adroit attempts to manage their complex lives through a flurry of activities and manipulations. Others fall into depressive responses. They come to see their lives as hopeless and cannot attend to even their basic human needs.

Of all the archetypal categories, false lovers are best suited to addiction model treatment. Their propensity to manifest a variety of addictive behaviors makes them good candidates for group therapy and treatment approaches that utilize a path of honesty and self-discovery outlined in twelve-step recovery programs such as Alcoholics Anonymous. This group is usually best understood and treated by addiction specialists and chemical dependency counselors. Their sexual acting out represents a facet of addictive disease as classically described in the "big book" of Alcoholics Anonymous (1976). This group commonly presents with a number of compulsive or addictive behaviors. Patients with addictive sexual disorders with prominent paraphilic features and those who meet the diagnostic criteria for a paraphilic disorder require additional treatment by experienced specialists in this field.

PROGNOSIS

The developmental task every false lover must face is to move from adolescent and hedonistic pursuits of self-gratification to a more mature and adult life in which the needs and feelings of others are given equivalent recognition and importance. They must also accept the need to live a life of rigorous honesty.

False lovers are usually professionally impaired by the time they come for assessment. Withdrawal from practice and intensive treatment are required, usually in an inpatient setting with peer professionals. Successful treatment and recovery require them to be rigorously honest, to overcome denial, to mature, and to develop increased compassion for others and commit to a lifelong recovery program.

Professional rehabilitation is possible after sufficient therapy and treatment, but by no means assured. Those who attain genuine recovery often do so through substantial personal change and spiritual awakening. Others comply with treatment and superficially express remorse and a desire to change, but harbor characterological pathology or impulse control disorders that cannot be overcome. This makes professional reentry unrealistic and hazardous. Recommendations from a multidisciplinary team of experienced professionals may be required.

11

The Dark King

If only it were all so simple! If only there were evil people somewhere insidiously committing evil deeds, and it were necessary only to separate them from the rest of us and destroy them. But the line dividing good and evil cuts through the heart of every human being. And who is willing to destroy a piece of his own heart?

> Alexander Solzhenitsyn, from William Miller, *Your Golden Shadow*, quoted in Zweig and Abrams 1991, p. v

The human devil resides in the pit of the belly. . . . Carnal pleasure is the main temptation the devil uses to lure the ego into the abyss of hell. Against this catastrophe the terrified ego strives to maintain control of the body at all costs. Consciousness, associated with the ego, becomes opposed to the unconscious or the body as the repository of the dark forces.

> Alexander Lowen, from William Miller, *Your Golden Shadow*, quoted in Zweig and Abrams 1991, p. 82

David Rayburn, a married, 30-year-old psychiatrist, was referred for assessment after a female patient complained to legal

authorities that he had touched her sexually in the course of
counseling her. Despite the patient's complaint and her testi-
mony against him in a subsequent criminal trial, David continued to believe that the sexual episode had been mutually
initiated and had heard caused no harm to the patient. In fact,
he maintained that within the context of a caring therapeutic relationship, the sexual touching had been of benefit to
the patient.

In the year after his assessment, he underwent a formal
hearing with the state licensure board. The findings included
not only legal violation and professional sexual misconduct, but
also conduct that was interpreted as professionally incompetent.
David unsuccessfully appealed these findings and the loss of
his license all the way to the state supreme court. He eventually
filed suit against the university residency program for inadequate training and supervision of him during his residency,
which he claimed caused his suffering and loss of license.

In the past, David had been attracted to other female
patients but claimed to have never sexually acted out his feelings. The patients who caught his attention had in common
a waif-like appearance and personality. They seemed to him
to be helpless and needy, and he perceived that they would
be grateful for any attention he would bestow on them. When
several of these women came forward with complaints of professional sexual misconduct characterized by inappropriate
verbal innuendoes and physical advances in the office, David
insisted they had conspired against him in an attempt to profit
from his misfortune after reading about his criminal trial in
the newspapers.

David grew up in a rigid, detached family, where discipline was strictly meted out and lines of responsibility were
clear. The emotion he became most comfortable expressing
was anger; fear, vulnerability, and emotional needs were bur-
ied deep inside. He married young, and he and his wife were
soon distant, duplicating the pattern in his childhood home.
Although he experimented with drugs and alcohol in college,
he had no problems with chemical use in adulthood, nor did

he evidence signs of sexual addiction or other compulsive or high-risk behaviors.

The Minesota Multiphasic Personality Inventory (MMPI-II) showed significant elevation on the psychopathy scale, and indicated the patient to be somewhat narcissistic and manipulative. He was not particularly anxious and showed no neurotic traits. Although David was young and immature, he was felt to have a more serious problem than simply lack of boundary education. Lacking significant Axis I pathology, his primary diagnosis was thought to be an Axis II personality disorder not otherwise specified (NOS) with prominent borderline and narcissistic features. David was judged to be professionally impaired, with a poor prognosis for returning to practice, and was advised to withdraw from medical practice and consider a change in career following psychotherapy treatment. He underwent a second-opinion assessment at another institution several months later. The findings were similar, with the additional diagnosis of narcissistic personality disorder.

Some men claim that they were born to become famous; others feel the mantle was imposed upon them. A common feature is that at some point in life, certain men come to believe that they have been bestowed with exceptional power and are destined to fulfill a call to action. It usually begins in childhood. The boy goes out in the world and tries to understand how his social system and society work, and how he may fit in. Along the way there are one or more defining events, wherein the boy discovers that others can exercise power, control, and manipulation in ways that hurt or control him. The lesson is not forgotten. The young man makes a vow not to become a victim of others, not to be dominated or used. He learns not to trust others and not to trust his emotions. He makes a vow to overcome his weaknesses and inadequacies, to become someone of power and significance. He not only identifies with the aggressor or exploiter who took advantage of him, but will supersede him in power and influence. This becomes his vision, his call to action.

This call or destiny becomes an organizing principle of his personal and professional life. It becomes the higher purpose, the raison d'être. The dark king is born when he interprets this call as an ordination. He comes to believe that this drive to succeed and acquire power and influence will become the dominant force in his life and the lives of those he comes to know.

Down through the centuries the model image of the helping professional has rested on oaths to remain the disinterested altruistic helper, concerned with those who are suffering in order to serve them. This is the light aspect of the work. Professional model images inherent in the physician, clergyman, and psychotherapist always contain a dark brother who is the opposite of the bright and shining ideal. The dark king uses his knowledge for his own personal profit. At best, he deceives himself along with those who are served, and at worst deceives only them. The dark king helps himself—through gains in prestige as well as financially—far more than he helps anyone who comes to him seeking assistance. He is not interested in the professional ethics and ideals of his profession; he fundamentally ignores his professional oath to work for himself, becoming the shadow professional. It is a shadow that may live in him or outside of him. Those he serves exert pressure on him to uphold his oath; yet he turns their personal vulnerabilities, conflicts, and problems into physical, emotional, spiritual, or legal issues that he alone can ameliorate. If they improve, he is the great healer; if they get worse, it is because they did not follow his directions properly (Zweig and Abrams 1990).

The dark king is driven by the desire to control and dominate. He believes he has earned the right to establish his rule, his dynasty, and to impose his vision, his will, upon his subjects. Many come to see themselves in possession of special insight and gifts.

Individuals who come into the world bearing superior talents, virtue, and knowledge are often rather isolated as children. They tend to be introverted, different, and intolerant of criticism and discipline, and they often become narcissistic. They prefer to develop relationships in which they are able to dominate or exercise more than equal power. The dark king often develops his charisma in association with his belief in a particular philosophy or school of thought. This often follows a period of adversity, painful transition, or personal distress. Others are attracted to the strength and intensity of his convictions, and perhaps to his ability to perform effectively professionally.

In coming to accumulate power, and in turn to be corrupted by it, dark kings often engage in sexual behavior that would be condemned as irresponsible in an ordinary person (Storr 1996). Characteristically, they do not see this as either the exercise of entitlement or as a manifestation of greed.

If there is one message to be conveyed about dark kings, it is that one should distrust those who hold power and are deeply self-absorbed and authoritarian. Those who preach of only one path to truth, whose oratory is powerful and leaves little room for debate, are particularly dangerous, especially those who appear to be paranoid (Storr 1996).

> We live in a time of critical excess. . . . In many of our lives these extremes take the form of symptoms: intensely negative feelings and actions, neurotic suffering, psychosomatic illnesses, depression, and substance abuse. . . . When we feel excessive desire, we push it into the shadow, then act it out without concern for others . . . through instant gratification or hedonistic activity, . . . in an uncontrolled drive for knowledge and power, . . . in a self righteous compulsion to help and cure others expressed in the distorted, codependent role of those in the helping professions, . . . in a desire to control our innately uncontrollable intimate lives, as expressed in narcissism, personal exploitation, manipulation of others, and abuse of women and children. [Zweig and Abrams 1990, p. xix]

The dark king initially experiences professional success and notoriety. Over time, while utilizing the resources at his disposal, he becomes more deliberate, cunning, and manipulative. Sexual exploitation becomes a right, an expression of power, of superiority, the imposition of dominance. Victims are carefully chosen to meet his needs and sexual agenda. He may be a Dr. Jekyll and Mr. Hyde figure with episodic acting out that appears superficially out of character. Or he may present as a refined persona with many friends and supporters who attest to his virtues and good moral character. He attempts to prove his innocence of wrongdoing, and explains personal and professional actions with refined justifications. Expect him to be therapy-wise, psychologically well-defended, and legally informed. Although dark kings are rare, they are the professional exploiters most frequently portrayed in the media. They are the evil sorcerers society fears may be lurking behind all sexually exploitative men. Once encountered and confronted, a dark king is not soon forgotten.

> "At midlife I met my devils. Much of what I had counted as a blessing became a curse. The wide road narrowed; the light grew dark. And in the darkness, the saint in me, so well nurtured and well coifed, met the sinner. . . . I had believed, with a kind of spiritual hubris, that a deep and committed inner life would keep me from human suffering, that it was managed with the discipline of self control. . . . My strengths began to feel like weaknesses, standing in the way of growth rather than promoting it. At the same time, dormant, unsuspected aptitudes awakened and arose rudely toward the surface, disrupting a self image to which I had become accustomed. . . . The thread of my life pulled; the story unraveled. And the ones I had despised and disdained were born in me—like another life, yet my life, its mirror image, its invisible twin. I could sense then why some people went mad, why some people had torrid love affairs despite a strong marriage bond, why some people with financial security began to steal or hoard money or give it all away. . . . I was capable of anything." [E. C. Whitmont, *The Symbolic Quest*, quoted in Zweig and Abrams 1991, p. 14]

Some dark kings present as disenfranchised, broken, and embittered. Through legal or organizational due process they have lost power. Over time they may be deposed and defamed, to be cast aside, left in abject spiritual poverty.

PATHOLOGIC NARCISSISM

For the dark king, professional sexual exploitation is a manifestation of narcissistic characterologic pathology. There are many definitions of narcissism. The one offered by Arnold Rothstein has particular value for the purposes of our discussion. He considers pathological narcissism to be an unrelenting, unrealistic pursuit of perfection. The term *narcissism* is derived from the clinical description (Narcisismus), offered by Paul Nacke in 1899 and Havelock Ellis in 1898, of a person who treats his own body in the same way in which some other sexual object would be treated to obtain complete gratification (Freud, in Morrison 1986). Yearnings for uniqueness, with regard to an idealized object, shame and humiliation over such yearnings, and the vulnerability that they engender (due to the danger of resistance, the denial of fulfillment, or a response of rejection or contempt from the object of desire) define an essential element in the narcissistic experience, according to Morrison. This aspect of narcissism is central to the experience of many dark kings.

Traumatic parental insensitivity or neglect, identification with parental grandiosity or narcissistic family systems, and constitutional aggressiveness may each play a part in the specific pattern of entitlement and exploitation of others developed by particular individuals, underscoring the need for careful assessment and strategic intervention on established defenses.

As Thomas Moore (1992) wrote, "Narcissism heals itself from loneliness into creation: in our narcissism we wound nature and make things that cannot be loved, but when our narcissism is transformed, the result is the love of self that engenders a sense of union with all of nature and things" (p. 74).

David Rayburn, whom we met at the beginning of this chapter, is representative of a relatively young "dark king" with significant characterologic pathology. He demonstrates an entire spectrum of narcissistic character defenses and elements of advanced disorder. The value system of narcissistic personalities is generally corruptible, in contrast to the doctrinaire morality of an obsessive-compulsive personality. The cold, calculating, predatory quality of their seduction and exploitation is in contrast with the warmer emotional quality of a hysteric caught in a neurotic conflict. Kernberg (1986) considers narcissism to be a continuum between adaptive character traits and defenses, through narcissistic personality, to narcissistic personality disorder, and on to narcissistic personalities with borderline features and the antisocial personality, which he sees as "an extreme form of pathological narcissism with a complete absence of an integrated superego" (p. 227).

> Oscar Jerman, a married, 40-year-old minister, became the subject of church inquiry when questions were raised regarding his use of church money for out-of-town activities. In the course of the investigations, allegations arose of sexual contact with a series of seven male parishioners and counselees, both adolescents and adults, over a six-year period of time. Oscar was referred for assessment because of these allegations. He denied some of the charges and justified and attempted to explain away some others. Eventually he admitted to sexually touching numerous parishioners, both with and without their consent. During his clinical assessment, he referred to himself as the victim of circumstances and events beyond his control. He neither voiced nor appeared to feel guilt or remorse. His regret for the professional sexual misconduct that transpired was largely based on the consequences for himself and his family.
>
> During Oscar's childhood, his father was distant, whereas his mother was controlling, demanding, and at times touched him inappropriately. He was a "perfect" child, and a high achiever in everything he tried. When Oscar was a teenager, he had been sexually molested by a priest repeatedly over a three-year period. When he married, his wife knew of his prior homosexual experiences but thought she could help him overcome the sexual abuse.
>
> Oscar's MMPI profile showed an individual who was immature, narcissistic, and self-indulgent. There was grandiosity and a tendency to blame others. His diagnoses were severe paraphilia (ephebophilia, which is pedophilia involving adolescents) as well as personality disorder NOS with dependent and antisocial traits. He was noted to have a chronic pattern

of exploitation, indicative of a sexual offender. He was advised to have no further contact with parishioners and to enter an inpatient sex offender treatment program.

Oscar's case points out the tendency for dark kings to come to the attention of regulatory agencies or other concerned parties because questions have arisen regarding types of power abuses other than sexual boundary violations. As Ross and Roy (1995) state:

> The more able, or cunning, or simply more polished and practiced seducer of clients has fewer probabilities of being unmasked than the inept, clumsy, or perhaps one-time culprit. This is the conclusion I have reached on the basis of my own experience. I have seen cases in which the activities of the expert and habitual seducers have finally been censured not because of their having been caught, but as a result of the discovery of other kinds of infractions that a growing and ever more careless sense of impunity had induced them to commit. The Greeks examined such occurrences with enormous psychological finesse and declared that great malefactors encountered the punishment of destiny not for their practice of good or evil actions, but for having given in to Hubris: arrogance, desiring too much, the recognition of no limits. It strikes me that professionals whom time will prove to be truly dishonest . . . are those who are possessed by hubris. [p. 48]

Gerald Zukosky, a married, 45-year-old physician, was referred by his medical licensing board for assessment in the wake of allegations of sexual exploitation of patients, which had resulted in criminal charges. Gerald admitted to sexual affairs over many years with dozens of patients, employees, co-workers, and other women in the community. He described the sense of power he had experienced in his sexual conquests but admitted to very little emotional involvement. He felt that the relationships had been consensual, even though he admitted to having used physical and verbal force, coercion, and manipulation in many cases. He systematically targeted a particular type of woman for pursuit, especially a vulnerable woman who would be unlikely to report him. Gerald appeared unable to understand that his affairs with patients constituted abuse of power.

In Gerald's family of origin, his father was physically and emotionally abusive, while his mother was dependent and compliant. His father had multiple extramarital affairs, which his mother felt she had no choice but to tolerate. When discussing his parents, Gerald could readily describe the abuse he experienced from his father, and the abuse his mother also suffered from him. He was unable to recall much at all about his relationship with his mother, whom he remembered as being passive, cold, and indifferent. Gerald was considered the favored son and had many privileges within the family. Becoming aggressive and hiding his own needs and vulnerability was the way to feel safe. Gerald became a powerful, controlling person who dominated those around him. He married a nurturing, caretaking woman, and rapidly lost sexual interest in her. Within months he initiated a series of extramarital affairs, which he expected his wife to accept.

During assessment, Gerald had very little insight into his behavior, and tended to rationalize, minimize, and justify his actions while blaming others. He seemed unable to imagine the impact of his behavior on the women with whom he had been sexual. Psychological testing supported an Axis II diagnosis of narcissistic personality disorder. He had no drug or alcohol dependency, but did meet the criteria for compulsive gambling.

Gerald's objectification and exploitation of women was felt to represent a paraphilia NOS with features of sexual perpetration, exploitation, and addiction. In addition to his narcissistic personality disorder, he had histrionic and antisocial personality traits. He was advised to withdraw from the practice of medicine, surrender his license, and enter an inpatient sex offender treatment program. It was considered unlikely that he could return to the practice of medicine.

Studies show that even one continuously sympathetic caregiver in childhood can make the difference between a seriously disturbed adult and someone who is emotionally healthy. Childhood experiences do trigger, and sometimes garble or distort, the love relationships made later. But nothing is cast in stone. As the child grows, he forges new attachments and some of these may dilute bad childhood experiences. This is an important conclusion, because it suggests that abused children may still be helped later in life.

Dark kings often have a long history of problems with impulse control and behavior disruptions, such as the expression of anger in the workplace. Their history of sexual misconduct tends to be deliberate and premeditated. Typically they are cool, calculating, and detached from those they employ, attend, and exploit. They are cunning enough to maintain appropriate boundaries in settings where they are under scrutiny, which makes it more difficult to believe that they would be exploitative. They are adept at manipulating colleagues and associates. They are skillful at using power and connections to fight allegations made against them. When caught, they may superficially be contrite, but will acknowledge only the unprofessional behavior that they believe is already known to others. When their manipulations are not successful in preventing personal consequences, they became narcissistically wounded. They often become hostile, engage in nasty counterattacks and threats, and are not fearful of damaging or hurting others, even those who are neutral or could potentially be sympathetic to their dilemma (Gonsiorek 1995).

PROGNOSIS

Dark kings are difficult to treat. Paraphilia, if present, is also difficult to treat. Addictive disease is relatively uncommon. Characteristically, their professional impairment is a risk to public safety and usually requires license suspension or revocation. Civil litigation and criminal prosecution is common. Treatment is prolonged and difficult, and is often not attempted until loss of licensure or incarceration. Most are unable to return to professional life.

The sociopathic and pathologically narcissistic professionals who exploit others consciously and without guilt or remorse are often perceived as criminals who will not be readily recognized by their colleagues and regulatory agencies, although they do continue to find new victims among the ill and helpless until they are finally stopped and appropriately disciplined. They deceive not so much those they are charged to serve and protect as much as themselves with their unconscious identity with their dark side, which Jung calls the shadow. They may experience healing or at least personal rehabilitation if they are able to look upon their exploitation with honesty, consciousness, and a genuine willingness to change. Addressing the professional shadow is of utmost importance.

However, there is danger here. The more individuated a man becomes, that is, the wider the realm of the unconscious spread out before him, the more powerful become the constellations of the unconscious. Acting in the unconsciousness means falling, over and over again, into one's own shadow.

The professional caught in the shadow lives more and more vicariously through those he is charged to serve and protect. Their gossip is his gossip; their friendships, love affairs, and sexual adventures become his experiences. He stops living his own life altogether. Those he serves are everything to him, his raison d'être. They live, love, and suffer for him, and he lives through them. Payment for services exists in order for us to live as decently as we deserve. The shadow holds veritable orgies with the concepts of transference and countertransference.

According to Diane Ackerman (1994),

> Nearly everyone who visits a therapist has a love disorder of one sort or another, and each has a story to tell—of love lost or denied, love twisted or betrayed, love perverted or shackled to violence. Broken attachments litter the office like pick-up sticks. People appear with frayed seams and spilling pockets. Some arrive pathologically disheartened by a childhood filled with hazard, molestation, and reproach. *Mutiles de guerre*, they are invisibly handicapped, veterans of a war they didn't even know

they were fighting. What battlefield could be more fierce, what enemy more dear? [p. 136]

Submerged or overt jealousy, insistence on increasing reliance on the professional in more and more aspects of life, resistance to any abrogation of our power, separation of the recipient of our desire from friends and acquaintances, and the devaluation of current and former lovers are all used to exert dominance and control. Adultery, for example, is not looked upon as a grave insult and aggression toward the marriage partner, but as a liberation from collective norms and an unsatisfactory mate. The dark king may play prophet by attempting to satisfy the religious needs of those he serves by pretending to transcendental wisdom. Every dream, every happening, event, illness, joy, grief, every accident experienced by the object of desire is interpreted and deduced for them in a manner than keeps them aligned to the will of the dark professional. . . . The shadow professional fails to recognize the dark hand of Moira [a Greek god associated with fate], to which even the gods, the unconscious must bow. [Sanford 1995, pp. 112–115]

The helping professional, whether a minister or not, is expected to have some spiritual principles. He is supposed to try, at least, to stand up with honesty and truthfulness for a definite way of life (a higher power) and service, either by virtue of a genuine relationship with God, or on the basis of his specially endowed gift of higher wisdom, and completion of a curriculum of study to obtain necessary knowledge to use for the benefit of others. The shadow aspect of this noble image of the spiritual professional is the hypocrite, who uses these principles not because he has faith, but because he wants to influence others, to wield power over them, and establish a social position that promotes the accumulation of status, wealth, or self-aggrandizement. The dark side of this intimate of God is the little lord almighty who is never at a loss for words or advice and who wants to represent himself to the world as well as to himself as better than he really is. The shadows of the false prophet, the hypocrite and the charlatan or quack accompany the helping professional all his life.

Helping professionals must work with their own psyches and shadows often without the aid of scientific data or constant professional supervision and helpful feedback. Our fundamental tools are ourselves, our honesty, our truthfulness, our intuition, and our own personal contact with the unconscious and the irrational. It is so human for us to represent these tools as better than they are and to fall into our professional shadow. We are too often pushed into the role of omniscience and possessor of infallible, divine knowledge. Neither we nor those we serve are willing to easily accept errors in judgment, imperfect memory, or unskillful words or action.

12

The Madman

When the [therapy] goes deep into the early and painful wounds and explores fearful places where madness threatens, the borderline enactments of the anima or animus figure emerge. They stand with a foot on either side of the borders between ego and archetype, reasonableness and passion, sanity and madness. They bring with them gusts of archetypal emotion as they put their finger on the precise spots of ego vulnerability. The danger looms of being emotionally overwhelmed.... When a person lacks relationship to others outside of the professional relationship, the situation can be much more tense. Reality seems to flourish only within the relationship. The urgency to live it right there becomes more compelling, and the sense of vulnerability all the more risky. Hidden in the urge for sexual gratification is purpose.

Ross and Roy 1995, p. 129

Lawrence Harrison was 50 years old when his licensing board requested an assessment after he had gotten into a fight with a colleague and caused him significant physical injuries. His colleague had accused him of having a sexual encounter with one of the clinic patients. Previously Lawrence had been reported to police by neighbors for an episode of domestic violence involving his wife. He had been known to verbally and physically abuse her and had assaulted other people in the hospital and at their country club as well. His behavior had resulted in several arrests as well as alienation from his family.

Lawrence stated that when he was a child his parents continually argued and called each other names. They were emotionally abusive to him as well. The only way he could get his parents' attention was to break dishes, kick or hit people, or slam doors.

By history and as observed by collateral sources of information, Lawrence had sudden and unpredictable changes in mood with a rapid onset of rage. He characteristically blamed others for the recurrent disruptive events of his life, and considered himself a victim of circumstances. Lawrence had experimented with marijuana in his youth, but was not using it at present. He did not meet the diagnostic criteria for a substance-related disorder.

Dr. Harrison was diagnosed as having bipolar disorder as well as narcissistic personality disorder and was considered impaired in his ability to practice medicine with safety. After a psychiatric hospitalization and the institution of pharmacotherapy, he was permitted to return to medical practice. Over the next several years there were occasional episodes of disruptive behavior. No further professional sexual misconduct or offense were alleged or reported.

Every professional begins his training and his career with a dream. The dream encompasses the career role that he may play in the future, the benefit his work will have for those he serves and for his society. It is one of the big dreams of life, and whether it is actually conceived in sleep or in a casual daydream, the image becomes a driving force in life. Without such a dream, a vision of becoming, few professionals could endure the rigors and demands of the work, the deprivation and hardship attendant with professional training.

However, life is often filled with unpredictable vicissitudes. On his journey, a professional may encounter a time of confusion, of torpor, or of disorder. Physical infirmities usually have some way of making us aware of their presence, and they are commonly met by our peers and families with compassion and sympathy. Mental disorders, however are more difficult to self-diagnose, accept, and address. The causes, as seen by different cultures, are summarized by Torrey (1986):

> Mental illness is universally thought to be caused by one of three things: biological events, experiential events, or metaphysical events. The first two are the foundation for Western therapy, the third for therapy elsewhere in the world. The difference is one of degree, however: all are found in some form in almost every culture in the world. Biological causes widely believed in by people in Western cultures include genetic damage, inborn constitutional factors, biochemical and metabolic imbalances, infections, drug toxicity and damage to the brain.... Experiential causes, especially experiences in childhood, are the hallmark of psychotherapy, and [treatment] consists of an exploration of these events.... Metaphysical causes are the most important ones in most of the world: the loss of the soul; the intrusion of a spirit into the body; sorcery; angering God. [pp. 25–26]

Madness (mental disorders) is at times a contributing factor to professional sexual misconduct and offense. Individual sufferers need treatment. Family members and concerned parties will seek to intervene in intolerable situations. Fear and uncertainty commonly arise. There are difficult questions to face. Can the affected individual (our archetypal madman) eventually regain his sanity and previous quality of life? Will he be able to function effectively as a person, and can he be trusted? Is he able to refrain from actions that would hurt him or others? Can his recovery be trusted to the point that we support his return to professional practice?

How we respond to these questions is not determined solely through medical model treatment, blood tests, brain scans, or response to psychotropic medication. How we contend with these questions the madman brings into our lives is determined by our personal experience and comfort in dealing with mental disorders, our social values and conventions, political considerations, and our motivation to assist a person with an illness that causes disability to be successful in returning to a meaningful and productive life. When we look at ourselves, we recognize our own mood swings, our anger and episodes of rage, our private disgusting or unusual thoughts, our own fears and anxieties, and our propensity for impulsive actions. We are uncomfortable with madness in part because at some level we know the enigmatic borderline between sanity and madness is sometimes hard to distinguish, and never far from any of us.

The madman archetype is categorized by the inconsistent and unpredictable nature of sexual impropriety, and the uncertain risk of recurrence. He has an erratic, unpredictable course in personal and professional life. At some point in his career, usually prior to allegations of sexual impropriety, he experiences significant difficulty functioning effectively, and seeks professional help. Sexual acting out occurs when management of the primary disorder is not optimal and is often associated with poor social judgment and loose professional boundaries. The dynamics of exploitation are often less ritualized, premeditated or easily defined. Usually, the professional does not meet the diagnostic criteria for psychosexual disorder or paraphilia. Sexual misconduct or offense is associated with disinhibition, lack of impulse control, cognitive distortion, dissociative state, psychotic thinking, or dementia.

In this typology, we are restricting the definition of the madman to those individuals who suffer from a mental dysfunction defined as an Axis I clinical disorder in the *DSM-IV*. Further, we are considering archetypes associated with professional sexual exploitation, so we would place those with a primary diagnosis of a sexual disorder or substance-related disorder in another archetypal category. Herein, the madman is one who suffers from a primary diagnosis of some other mental disorder that is considered a significant contributing factor to professional sexual exploitation. The differential diagnosis of such disorders is found in Chapter 3. The most common diagnoses are major depression with psychotic features, bipolar affective disorder, atypical psychosis, dissociative disorder, and organic mental disorders associated with medical conditions of unknown etiology. Chemical dependency is a common complicating problem. Treatment is often initially effective, and the professional may perform well for periods of time. Some, however, will have reactivation of their primary disorder, and as their madness intervenes, the professional may be discovered to have again engaged in sexual impropriety in either his personal or professional life.

Lawrence Harrison exemplifies the professional whose behavior is intermittently out of control because of an Axis I psychiatric disorder. When Lawrence was in his third and fourth decades of life, he would have laughed if he had been told that he suffered from a significant affective disorder. He was aware that he had times when he felt emotion and mood intensely, but he believed that he was not significantly different from other family members or friends. Like many with bipolar disorder, he liked many features of his hypomanic episodes. He was very productive during these times, gregarious, and filled with energy and ideas. His behavior, while erratic and somewhat unpredictable, was held in check when it began to create concern for others.

For decades the advantages of his mood swings seemed to outweigh the disadvantages. However, as consequences began to impact upon his personal life, he did began to wonder why he was different in some ways from others. He believed that his medical knowledge would come to his aid and would protect him from an undiagnosed illness. He thought he would be able to make any necessary self-diagnosis without the help of others. His bipolar affective disorder finally became strong enough to overcome his defenses, and for a long period of time he denied he was ill and resisted attempts to diagnose and treat his disorder.

Today Lawrence is more realistic about his own infirmities. He has come to recognize the value of seeking out and accepting the opinions of others regarding his conduct and affect. He has learned how to cope with his chronic disorder. Several cycles of mania and depression have ensued since initial diagnosis and treatment. He is now grateful that he can practice medicine at all, and has come to have much more compassion for the mentally ill. Living with the difficulties and stigma of a disorder that can cause symptoms without warning or a clear exacerbating cause is a humbling experience, even for the proudest man.

William Benedict was 41 years old when he was referred by the state medical licensure board to the professional assessment program with allegations of professional sexual misconduct. Married for seven years, he and his wife had chosen not to have children. He was working as a pediatric infectious disease specialist at a large teaching hospital affiliated with a major university. Concerns had been raised about his behavior toward some young male teenagers in his practice, as he spent unusual amounts of time with certain patients and their families. He had a particular interest in AIDS and treatment-related problems in male adolescents. Concern was raised regarding the nature of his relationship with several of these young men.

William categorically denied sexual involvement with any of his patients. In the course of the assessment he became withdrawn and despondent. On the third day he admitted to his assessment physician that he had become intrigued with the prospect of developing AIDS himself. Secretly, he had confiscated HIV-contaminated needles and had injected himself with them on at least four different occasions.

Psychological testing and psychiatric diagnostic interviews confirmed a diagnosis of a major dissociative disorder. He was hospitalized in a psychiatric facility that specialized in the treatment of this disorder. After seven weeks his condition stabilized, and he returned to his home to begin outpatient therapy. Over the next six months he gradually improved. William slowly came to terms with his mental disorder, and after more than two years was able to return to academic medical research on a limited basis. About three years after the initial assessment, he contacted the assessment program and indicated that he was working as a clinical instructor for a medical school. He and his wife had decided to adopt a child. He had never become HIV positive, reaffirmed that he had used HIV-infected sharps to inject himself, and was now thankful that he had never developed AIDS.

William reminds us that there are many ways in which our professional–patient relationships directly and profoundly affect our own lives. As his career in academic medicine and research advanced, he became particularly intrigued with families living with a member who had developed AIDS. He had become deeply emotionally connected with the lives of young men who were facing terminal illness and death. This identification was more unconscious than conscious, submerged in part through the rationalization and justification that he was engaging in scientific inquiry and research. Yet this intrigue became in its own way a kind of nonsexual voyeurism, in which he sought out the more subtle details of the lives and feelings of the tragedy each young patient faced. As Susan Sontag so eloquently described in her powerful and erudite books *Illness as Metaphor* (1995) and *AIDS and Its Metaphors* (1989), intellectual and erotic attitudes, known as "romantic agony," can be derived from chronic illnesses lived vicariously by a sensitive person. A person dying young is viewed as living out a fated romantic tragedy. The ultimate identification is to seek out the opportunity to join the afflicted in the illness, the suffering, the love-death.

PROGNOSIS

Prognosis depends on precise and appropriate diagnosis and ongoing effective treatment. Treatment of medical or psychiatric disorders is required to appreciate the natural history of the problem and make cogent recommendations concerning the staging and safety of professional reentry. Lack of compliance with prescribed medication, the use of mood-altering substances, or the failure to continue in monitoring of medication and ongoing therapy are the most common preventable factors associated with further professional sexual misconduct or offense. Return to practice is possible if the professional undergoes successful treatment and complies with ongoing therapy, medication (if needed), structured practice boundaries, and a continuing-care contract.

Part III

Healing the Wounded

13

The Forgotten Victims: The Offender's Family

All the facts of the following story, which received wide media coverage, are real; only the names have been changed to protect the privacy of the persons involved.

At age 26, Bill, a junior high school science teacher, became infatuated with Cindy, one of his students. At the end of the school year, shortly after Cindy's fourteenth birthday, Bill and the girl became sexual. The consequences of Bill's sexually exploitative behavior forever changed the lives of his family.

Raised in a very strict, conservative Baptist home, Bill's wife Colleen was brought up to focus her attention on her husband and his career. She made a perfect match for Bill, who soon was making local headlines for his innovative programs in the classroom. After the beginning of her third pregnancy Colleen began to feel that something was wrong with her husband. He seemed preoccupied, spent an excessive amount of time at school after hours, and received many calls from students at home. Shortly after classes ended that summer, Bill ran away with Cindy, intending to establish a new life in another state. A nationwide manhunt with widespread publicity ensued.

When Bill was arrested weeks later and sentenced to twelve years' imprisonment without possibility of parole, Colleen was forced into an escalating crisis management mode. Their home was eventually foreclosed, health insurance for the third child's delivery was canceled, and all available money disappeared. Colleen was hounded by the media and felt bound by her religious beliefs to publicly commit to a marriage to a man whose behavior was absolutely abhorrent to her.

Overnight Colleen's financial status changed from being a middle-class housewife to a poverty-stricken single mother of three, living in her parents' home. She got a crash course in Welfare 101, spending hours on buses going to appointments with a constantly changing array of case workers, waiting on line to get free food for her children, and worrying about where to obtain clothes and other necessities for the family. Previously a firm believer in financial independence, she felt humiliated by the necessity to accept handouts from her church, parents, and friends. Devastating to her self-esteem was going from adult independence to being once again treated like a child, and she was criticized by her parents for her poor choice of husband.

Recognizing the need to support herself, Colleen obtained scholarships to attend college, eventually earned a graduate degree, got off welfare after several years, and became a self-supporting career woman. She continued to visit her husband weekly at the prison, and worked hard to keep her children connected to him. All the skills Colleen had used to assist her husband in his career as a teacher became focused on balancing her education, her marriage, and her children.

Colleen's pastor was firmly against divorce. The secular community, on the other hand, gave her no support for staying in the marriage, and, in fact, considered her bizarre for making this choice. She felt a great deal of shame, and chose to keep her situation secret from most people. With her husband in prison, she felt it would be unfair to let him experience the full extent of her anger. She sublimated the rage she felt about the betrayal and about the changes in her life plans by focusing on her career and her children.

Colleen arranged for a counselor to visit Bill at the prison, and she also participated in some joint sessions. Eventually he fully acknowledged the damage he had caused to both 14-year-old Cindy and to his own family, worked through his own childhood abandonment issues, became a very involved father via phone calls and letters, and waited for the opportunity to be a committed and involved partner to Colleen. Colleen, on the other hand, had barely begun to heal from the betrayal, in part because Bill's lengthy prison sentence prevented them from working through critical personal issues. She had also lost the ability to trust her own decision-making skills, nor did she take the time to nurture herself.

Colleen's three children grew up with ongoing emotional support from their grandparents and the church community. Ten years later, they were doing well in school and emotionally, but Colleen was still angry, still struggling with many unresolved feelings about what had happened, very ambivalent about her husband, and still waiting for his release in the year 2000 and hoping they could somehow get their life back in order. She admitted she had long since lost her faith in her church and in the principles with which she had been raised. She still considered herself as much a victim of her husband's behavior as was the young girl he'd molested.

She now struggles with intensive and delayed anger responses that are easily triggered by what would appear to be unrelated events. Both Bill and Colleen recognize that this may be a very difficult barrier to the recovery of their marriage.

When sexual exploitation comes to light and a crisis ensues, attention is immediately focused on two people—the exploitative professional and the victim (or victims). Yet there is usually another person whose life has been adversely affected by the exploitation, but who is generally forgotten—the spouse or significant other of the exploitative professional. In the best-case scenario, the offending professional is assessed, enters primary treatment, and will remain out of professional practice for an extended period of time. If he is committed to the process, he receives support and advocacy from his helpers, and he is introduced to other professionals who have been exploitative and have recovered. He emerges from his experience with a whole new support system and an increased sense of self-worth. A less favorable outcome might include a permanent loss of his license, and perhaps even a prison term.

No matter what the outcome, the partner is significantly affected in many ways. But unlike the offender, there is frequently no one, or only a few people, to support and advocate for her. Typically very little attention is paid to her needs, and she usually goes through an enormous personal, emotional, and financial crisis, alone and unsupported. Her needs are not attended to, and she is often cast in a supportive role for the offender and becomes a pillar of strength for their children. This chapter addresses the issues that arise when clinicians who are working with impaired professionals and their families need to understand the experience of the spouse or partner so as to be able to better help the entire family.

Traditionally, being the wife of the doctor or minister was a career in itself. Supporting her husband's profession both publicly and privately was the wife's full-time occupation. Inevitably, much of her self-esteem came from her husband's profession and the respect with which he was treated. In the aftermath of the disclosure of his sexual misconduct, her entire identity feels threatened, and her self-worth crumbles. When the wife's education and skills have allowed her to work together with her husband, once he is dismissed or loses his license, she too can no longer continue to work in the field. A complete career change must be made in the midst of high anxiety and feelings of worthlessness.

Often her lifestyle and financial status were also dependent on his career. If he was a minister, the house she lived in may have belonged to the parish and been part of his career benefits. Even if she had her own career, her husband's income and position in the community were usually very important to her.

In any committed relationship, disclosure of sexual impropriety creates an immediate personal crisis for the wife or partner. Although individuals react differently, most significant others experience shock, denial, fear of abandonment, assumption of guilt and responsibility for the problem, anger over the betrayal, and finally gradual healing. These stages take place whether or not the couple stays together.

In the case of the wife of a minister, when the crisis of disclosure of her husband's misconduct first comes to light, she goes through all the above reactions, but in addition has other factors to contend with. Her husband's misconduct often is made public, and her reaction is closely observed—by the congregation and the neighbors. It is traditional for the wife to "stand by her man" in such situations; there are many recent examples from the world of politics, even in cases where sexual exploitation was not involved: Hillary Rodham Clinton going on TV with her husband in 1992 to demonstrate solidarity with him and save his candidacy after a past affair came to light, and again standing by his side in 1998 during his presidency when an alleged sexual relationship with a young White House intern came to light; the wife of presidential advisor Dick Morris on the cover of *Newsweek* with her husband a week after his affair with a prostitute was revealed (the Morrises were divorced soon thereafter); presidential candidate Gary Hart's wife sticking by her husband in 1984 after pictures of him on a boat with a young woman on his lap were plastered over the covers of the tabloids.

The professional's wife typically plays out this scenario no matter what her inner turmoil. Later, she may experience additional anger over having been "forced" to assume this role. Colleen, the wife of the teacher who was imprisoned for sexual misconduct, reported, "Those of us with a traditional religious upbringing, who are homemakers married to a professional man, have a much higher profile and an active role in the church. Our position forces us to display a 'correct' response dictated by our belief

system, with often a simultaneous loss of faith in that same belief
system."

Another factor for professional spouses is often their very real
financial dependence on their husbands. A doctor may need to
take extended time off from his medical practice; a minister may
lose his pastoral job and the home that came with it; a psychotherapist may lose his practice—all these economic consequences can
be very frightening to the wife, especially if she is not herself a
significant wage earner. The professional may have been diverting
income to his extramarital relationship activities. Said one wife, "My
husband funded his relationship with money he had withdrawn
from his retirement fund without my knowledge. This later came
to light when our taxes were audited for that year for failure to
report this 'income.' "

Add to this the cost of psychological assessment and therapy
for the misconduct, legal costs of defending himself against lawsuits arising from his misconduct, and the recent decisions by
medical and psychological malpractice insurance carriers to exclude
from malpractice coverage the cost of fighting sexual misconduct
lawsuits, and it is evident that there are many financial costs to the
family of the husband's sexual misconduct. Given this reality, divorce may seem an unrealistic option.

SHAME, BLAME, AND KEEPING SECRETS

When a professional is sent for assessment and/or treatment following the revelation of some sexual misbehavior, the partner is
left at home to face the fallout of the impropriety alone. In the
early stages of treatment, impaired professionals are often allowed
minimal phone calls home. The children wonder what has happened, and it is up to the spouse to decide how much to tell them.
At this early stage, the decision is often to say as little as possible,
even if the children are themselves adults.

Early on, spouses of exploitative professionals often experience
profound shame. Their husbands have had sexual relations outside
of their marriage, and a common reaction is to wonder "what's

wrong with me?" Blaming oneself for a partner's affairs or need for some sexual expression outside the marriage is natural. Added to this is the fear that others will draw the same conclusion. The spouse's shame is intensified when the offender was considered a role model for moral behavior, as clergymen and helping professionals generally are. Additional shame results from the community's tendency to see the professional and his wife as a team, and therefore to tar the wife with the same brush. As the shame intensifies, the spouse's tendency is to keep quiet rather than seek support, and to put up a good front.

The wife is often seen by the victim, by the media, and by the professional's clients, patients, or parishioners as part of the problem, an extension of the perpetrator, rather than for what she really is—a secondary victim. She is often blamed and shamed. Spouses of exploitative ministers have related being ostracized by their congregation because of their husband's behavior. At the very time that the wife most needs a support system, her community tends to cut her off and isolate her. Her only support, in fact, seems to be her husband.

Legg and Legg (1995) wrote about ministers' families, "When male clergy acted out sexually, all of the wives reported that church gossip labeled them as frigid, inadequate women or as spoiled, self-centered children. This occurs, we believe, because some simply cannot blame their minister; therefore his wife must be at fault. The wife, who has already been a victim of her husband's betrayal, now becomes the victim of a second betrayal by members of the congregation" (p. 147).

The wife often loses support from her family of origin as well. This description relates to wives of exploitative clergymen:

> Shame . . . extended to many of the families of origin, especially if they were active and devout members of their churches. Wives most often felt blamed by both their own parents and their spouse's parents. They either were not adequate as wives or they shouldn't have married these men in the first place. They got very little support for staying in the marriage. If they divorced, they were often shamed for their lack of moral fiber. If they

became emotionally or financially dependent on their parents,
they were treated like incompetent children. Several reported
losing relationships with their siblings and extended families.
[Legg and Legg 1995, p. 147]

Often a family will choose to help a daughter only under certain circumstances dependent on their belief system, for example, only if she divorces her husband, or alternatively, only if she stays with him.

There is also often an immediate reassessment of the relationship between the professional's parents and his partner. To choose between a son and a daughter-in-law is not a choice a parent wants to make; yet often that choice determines whether they will have continuing contact with grandchildren. Fear of losing the relationship with their grandchildren may be a greater concern than the conduct of their own child or the impact on the spouse. The crisis may additionally lead to discovery of information that had been kept secret in the family—that the exploitative professional had been in psychological treatment as a teenager, that there is a family history of alcoholism, or that a relative had engaged in inappropriate sexual actions in the past. These secrets may serve to compound the wife's feelings of betrayal and increase her anger.

Faced with the knowledge of her husband's betrayal, compounded by isolation from the community, the spouse's fears of abandonment from childhood become reactivated at this time. To protect herself, she may view this as the time to fight for the survival of her marriage and her lifestyle by suppressing her own needs, fears, and anger, and actively supporting her husband, rather than asking for the emotional support that she so badly needs at this time. For example, the wife may be too invested in protecting her husband to be willing to open up and reveal their real problems and marital difficulties, much less her own negative feelings, during family sessions in treatment.

When the exploitative professional's behavior has resulted in legal problems, the spouse is likely to be questioned intensely by the authorities. Most spouses do not realize their right to legal counsel even if being questioned by a medical licensing board.

Minimizing any problems and downplaying any actions that might tend to support a finding of guilt ties tightly into direct survival needs of the relationship and the ability to get by after the consequences are determined.

Under intense questioning and the expectation that the partner should have the answers, the spouse comes to feel even less competent in her ability to make decisions.

The spouse may deflect her anger onto the treatment team, the interventionist, or the corporation. At times she may accurately perceive that the treatment team wants to use her as a source for the information her husband has been unwilling to reveal. Clinicians need to examine their ethical responsibilities, and weigh their responsibility to protect the public as well as to protect the spouse, family, and identified patient.

It is very helpful if someone from the treatment team calls and supports the spouse, listens to her feelings of the moment, explains why her husband cannot contact her much, and encourages her to write down her thoughts and feelings and see a counselor. This person can also help the spouse sort out options for talking with the children about their father's problem and providing them with information that is appropriate to their developmental stage.

DISCLOSURE

While publicly engaged in damage control and in presenting a united front, while supporting her husband as effectively as possible in order to hasten his return to their previous life (not necessarily their real life, but at least their life as she believed it was), what is the wife actually feeling? Her initial feelings depend on the nature of the disclosure. Some variables are:

- Was everything revealed at the first disclosure?
- Was there a sudden disclosure, or did she have ongoing suspicions or knowledge?
- Was the initial disclosure public or private? Private disclosure gives the couple some time to sort out their feelings, whereas public disclosure forces public statements and in-

stant feedback and opinions from others. On the other
hand, private disclosure tends to force the spouse to maintain the secret even from her own children, whereas public
disclosure brings it all out in the open, which can result in
greater criticism but also unexpected support.

The nature and amount of the disclosure to the partner can
have a long-lasting impact on the couple's relationship.

John, a 32-year-old gynecologist, had had a series of affairs with
patients. His wife, Jodie, was unaware of this until one patient
complained to John's medical licensing board, and an article
about the complaint appeared in the local paper. John told
Jodie that the charges were untrue, that this was a disgruntled
patient who had made up the story in order to get back at
him for some imagined wrong. Jodie fully supported John,
arguing vehemently on his behalf with friends who suggested
that there might be a basis for the charges. Over the next few
weeks she devoted herself fully to John's defense, convinced
of his innocence, in the meantime alienating her family and
friends who thought she was probably deluding herself.

   Two months later when John appeared before the medical board, Jodie insisted on accompanying him; she was sure
he would be vindicated. At the hearing, she found the alleged
victim's story very persuasive, and was shocked to hear of
multiple allegations against him involving other patients. At
the end of the hearing, John's license was suspended. Jodie
went home feeling intense anger and betrayal, not only at
John's initial betrayal by being sexual with patients, but even
more at the lying that had gone on since the first newspaper
article. She felt tremendous shame over her gullibility, and
could barely face her family and friends, who had been right
all along.

   John eventually went to treatment for chemical dependency and sexual addiction, became actively committed to recovery, and was able to resume practicing medicine, although

not gynecology. Jodie, however, was never able to forgive the double betrayal and the couple divorced.

Disclosure is usually a process rather than a one-time event. Much of the time, the identified patient does not tell all at first, then comes back to reveal more. This sequence further erodes the partner's trust; it can be helpful for couples to understand that initial full disclosure is the exception rather than the rule. It is unfortunately all too common for exploitative professionals to initially minimize their misconduct, not only to licensing boards and assessment teams but also to their spouses. This is probably less likely in the case of naive princes and wounded warriors than in the other archetypes, although there are as yet no data on this. What is clear, however, is that when a wife who has actively supported her husband because she believed in his innocence eventually learns that he continued to lie to her about the allegations after they were made public, the damage and sense of betrayal is compounded, and healing is that much more difficult.

Legg and Legg (1995) write about a sexually exploitative clergyman:

> In another instance, the wife told everybody she could reach in the congregation that her husband was "no sexual addict" and would never betray her. He already had admitted to officials that he had crossed the sexual boundaries in his present and past congregations. He had not told the wife, nor had the officials. Not until she was confronted with details and her husband's admission six months later did she stop contacting parishioners. In addition to the betrayal she now had to deal with the humiliation of her denial and of her telephone calls. We believe it is important for the spouse to not only be told of the charges immediately but to be constantly informed of the evidence as it becomes known and to be helped in accepting the truth. [p. 150]

No matter how and when disclosure takes place, the spouse will experience pain. However, early disclosure and a willingness to answer her questions honestly and provide as much information

as she wants are factors that will make it more likely that the relationship will survive the crisis. A therapist can help facilitate this
process.

LOSS OF SELF-ESTEEM, USE OF ANGER, AND
GETTING STUCK IN THE VICTIM ROLE

Before disclosure, the offender's spouse often has some suspicions,
but tends to believe her husband (who discounts and explains away
her suspicions) rather than her own intuition. As a result she comes
to distrust her ability to monitor events, and later often says, "I
thought I was going crazy." The offending spouse supports this
illusion to cover his own behavior. One exploitative psychiatrist
encouraged his wife to get psychiatric help to deal with her suspicions and depression, and referred her to one of his own trusted
colleagues. When the truth comes out, the wife may experience
relief, "I am *not* going crazy."

On the other hand, if the spouse was unaware of the exploitation until the crisis or disclosure, she is likely to begin to question her grasp of reality. "How could I not have known this was
happening?" "How much of my life with him was a lie?" "I must
be a laughingstock at the office." "What must those women he had
sex with think of me?" "How could I have thought everything was
fine?" "There must be something wrong with me." However, generally the crisis of the moment precludes opportunities for her to
reveal and process her feelings.

Instead, the disbelief is soon replaced by numbness and the
wife is forced to pick up the pieces of her life. Caring for the children becomes an important occupation, especially if the husband
is away for weeks or months for treatment. Her feelings are stifled
while she gives emotional support to her husband, with the goal
of keeping the family together. Her career outside the home, if
she has one, becomes an important source of family income, and
a good avenue of escape from her feelings and worries. The organizational skills that were so useful to her as a minister's wife or a
doctor's wife now are dedicated to providing a "normal" life for

herself and her children. Crisis management is the most urgent
need. Her feelings of low self-esteem come and go, intermixed with
a sense of competence as she engage in damage control.

According to Colleen, the woman whose husband went to
prison for having sex with a 14-year-old student, "Survival became
measured in 'effectiveness,' not in how I am feeling today. Crisis
management became the pattern of reaction . . . . I was never able
to catch up and get control of the runaway train. For years, my
anger was a channeled energy source. It was unfocused, but it kept
me going."

The children, too, react in various ways. Some move into the
"perfect child" role in order to help Mom out. Others begin to
act out and cause problems, so as to deflect attention from the
identified patient, their father. Dealing with the children puts additional stress on the mother.

Some wives may remain in the denial stage for months, due
to lack of support, fear for their safety, or inability to deal with
the possible loss of the relationship. For most spouses, however,
as the crisis mode recedes, anger will eventually come to the surface. Depending on the offender's behavior before and after the
disclosure, on the disruption in her life resulting from the offense
and the disclosure, on the support and counseling she may have
received during the early months, and on her own unresolved family of origin issues, her anger may be immense and long-lasting.

When Linda married Barry, he was a 40-year-old internist with
five children from an earlier marriage and a very successful
medical practice in a small town. The couple had two more
children within three years, and Linda was a very committed
housewife and mother, caring for her two children as well as
caring part-time for the two youngest children from Barry's
previous marriage. He had been married when he met Linda
and initiated an affair with her, but she accepted his explanation that his wife was impossible to get along with. Barry was
the pillar of the community, highly respected, and very active
in his church. He was clearly the moral leader at home, with
rigid and definite attitudes on how things should be done.

After five years of marriage, Barry was sent for assessment when a patient complained that he had been sexual with her. What came to light was that Barry had a long history of affairs with patients, office staff, and hospital personnel. A "self-serving martyr," he went through months of minimization of his problems and self-serving justifications to his wife before recognizing the severity of his problem and becoming seriously committed to recovery. Primary treatment for sex addiction and subsequent rehabilitation took a year, after which his medical license was restored with stipulations, and he took a salaried job at a much lower income and with much less prestige than his previous situation.

Linda supported Barry through the first rough year. She stoically went through the move to a smaller house, kept up a good front to her family and his when he was expelled from his church community, and protected the kids from hearing anything bad about their father. She had grown up in a rigid, disengaged religious family where one "did the right thing," ignoring one's feelings. She felt thoroughly victimized by her current situation, but declined to talk to anyone about it. Her anger seethed just below the surface. She was unwilling to consider trusting Barry again. After a year she reluctantly agreed to accompany Barry to a weekend for couples recovering from sex addiction, but could not deviate from her victim stance and her anger. She did not accept a recommendation to get counseling because she believed that the only person in the family with a problem was Barry. Barry believed that she needed more time and decided to simply accept her anger, and, in fact, after two more years the relationship began to improve.

Linda's healing from the trauma of Barry's sexual offenses was markedly delayed because of her difficulty moving away from the victim stance and her belief that people should be able to work out their problems by themselves. In contrast, the outcome for the relationship can be better and recovery quicker when there is full disclosure to the spouse and early acceptance of responsibility by the offender, when communication is good, when both partners are active in the recovery process, and when they can make some meaning out of the experience, as demonstrated by the next case:

> Lawrence was a 55-year-old minister, married to Sandy for 30 years, when his church board fired him after learning that he had initiated a sexual relationship with a parishioner while counseling her regarding her marital problems. When news of Lawrence's transgression became public, two other parishioners came forward and described prior affairs with him. The church board gave Lawrence and his wife two weeks to move out of the parish-owned home; the congregation ostracized Sandy, who had been actively involved in church leadership for many years.
>
> Sandy was taken completely by surprise by Lawrence's affairs. She initially experienced fear, betrayal, shame, and a sense of unreality about her perception of the world. Lawrence viewed his bottoming out as a wake-up call, an opportunity to get help, change his life, and be able to respect himself again. He obtained counseling and became active in a twelve-step program for sex addiction. He initiated long discussions with Sandy, fully disclosing to her what he had done and accepting responsibility for the pain he was causing her. She was able to express her anger to him. Sandy went to counseling as well, and was able to talk about her sense of betrayal, her anger, and her difficulty coping with the loss of community support and her change in lifestyle.
>
> Sandy and Lawrence moved to a different city, where she got a job as a kindergarten teacher and he took up carpentry. Rebuilding their marriage was a high priority for both. Eventually they began counseling couples recovering from sex addiction.

The adverse consequences experienced by the spouse of a sexually exploitative professional may be as great as the consequences to the offender. When a married person engages in extramarital sex, the partner who learns about it feels betrayed and victimized. The sense of being a victim is even greater for the exploitative professional's spouse who additionally experiences financial loss, being blamed along with the offender, and loss of community respect and prestige. She truly is a victim. However, the depth of the feelings of betrayal and victimization are influenced not only by the current events such as the perpetrator's behavior and community response, but also by the wife's experiences in her family of origin. If she was betrayed and victimized in childhood as a result of physical or sexual abuse, or if she was physically or emotionally abandoned by a parent, then her reaction is likely to be magnified.

Colleen (discussed above) wrote, "If the professional has broken the law, the legal system also wants the spouse to take the victim stance. Only then is she granted some respect and help; otherwise she is treated with less respect than the offender himself—she is given no answers, no counsel, and no knowledge of what could happen and what alternatives are available, such as separation of community property, restoration of her former name, or other actions that might ease her ability to function post-crisis."

To be a victim is to be disempowered. To be able to make real choices, including forgiving the offender and choosing to leave, or to stay in the marriage, the wife needs to move beyond the victim role, and to move through and beyond anger. Victims do not have the power to make real choices; they can only react.

Victims are also at risk of becoming victimizers. In the case of the betrayed spouse who cannot move beyond the victim stance, one possible coping strategy is to turn to one of her children for nurturing. This child becomes her confidant, her support, the person she leans on. The child then may become a victim of "emotional incest," subsequently at high risk for his or her own addictions and psychopathology. Awareness of this potential trap may help the distressed spouse to avoid it, seeking support instead from peers and professionals.

The children of exploitative professionals are at high risk themselves. For at least several months they essentially lose both parents, one in reality (if in treatment or in prison) and the other emotionally. The offender's spouse may be afraid to love for fear of the inevitability of being hurt. The personality characteristics in her children that are "just like Daddy," which she used to find charming, now drain her, with the fear of just how much like Daddy they might be. Ways of preventing the child from feeling overly responsible for the family problems include honest discussion rather than keeping family secrets, and complete acceptance of responsibility by the offender for his actions.

REENTRY

Impaired professionals who are sent for treatment are often out of the home for several months. During this time many changes take place. The spouse and children may find that they have done much better without Dad than they expected—the peace and quiet of not having to deal with his problems may have been an unexpected benefit. Wives who did not know how to change a tire or adjust the hot water heater may have discovered or developed new skills and competencies. Their relationships with their children may have improved.

When the father returns home, he may have to reenter the family in a different role. Treating clinicians need to make the patient aware of this possibility. Family members may be torn between feeling glad he's back and feeling angry. To prepare the entire family, it can be helpful for the professional to have one or two therapeutic leaves to go home during a lengthy treatment process.

THE STAGES OF RECOVERY FOR THE SPOUSE OR SIGNIFICANT OTHER

The spouse who finds herself stuck in the role of victim can benefit from therapy as well as involvement in a twelve-step support group. This help will facilitate her moving through the stages of her own recovery, which in some ways parallel the stages of recovery for the exploitative professional described in the next chapter.

Carnes (1991) identified six developmental stages in the recovery of the sexual coaddict: the development stage, crisis/deci-
sion stage, shock stage, grief stage, repair stage, and growth stage.
Although not all exploitative professionals are sexually addicted and
not all their wives are coaddicts, these stages provide a good description of the process through which the offender's spouse moves
in her path of recovery. The spouse may move through these stages
at different tempos and at different times from the addict, so that
the two partners may be out of sync for the first few months.

In the *development stage*, according to Carnes, despite growing awareness of the problem, denial persists, resulting at times in
outrageous behavior. During this stage the wife may have some idea
that there is a problem, particularly if allegations of sexual misconduct have been made against her husband, but her denial may be
strong, especially if the offender colludes in denying what happened.

The *crisis stage* leads to greater awareness and a commitment
to change. The wife can no longer deny that a real problem exists. For the professional's spouse, the crisis stage is usually accompanied by fear—fear of abandonment, fear of loss of community
and family support, fear of economic insecurity.

The *shock stage*, a period of emotional numbness, comes next.
This is the period during which the wife buries her feelings and
concentrates on providing support for her husband and on presenting a united front with him.

In the *grief stage*, denial collapses and the full impact of the
losses is grasped, resulting in intense pain. Feelings of grief are
usually preceded by anger, which is essential for healing. If the
spouse cannot or will not feel her anger and then express it, forgiveness will be very difficult. Forgiveness is facilitated when the
offender is willing to hear the spouse's anger and acknowledges
his responsibility in causing her hurt and anger.

As part of this stage, the spouse grieves the loss of her life as
it used to be. In addition to the obvious losses that the wife of the
offender must contend with (economic losses, loss of prestige and
community standing, loss of her role as the respected professional's

wife), there is a deeper loss—the loss of her spouse as she had believed him to be and the loss of the reality of her life as she had perceived it to be. She has learned that her husband had lied to her about many things, that he was leading a Jekyll and Hyde existence, that her trust in him had been misplaced. She must accept the likelihood that in the future other past falsehoods will be revealed.

The *repair stage*, an intense period of personal growth and renewal, which impacts on the relationship, follows. In this stage, work on family-of-origin issues can be very helpful. The woman recognizes her childhood losses, sees in which ways she is trying to get her unmet childhood needs met in her current relationships, and sorts out what is realistic and what is not. In this stage she learns to separate her behaviors and their consequences from those of her spouse's, that she is not responsible for his behavior and cannot change him. She unties her self-esteem from her husband's actions and from his behavior toward her. If he was her higher power before, she recognizes that her self-worth must come from within, and she focuses on understanding and expressing her own needs and preferences. In this stage, too, she learns to set appropriate boundaries about which behaviors are or are not acceptable within the relationship,

Finally, in the *growth stage*, which begins about two years into recovery, the spouse or significant other has developed an inner core of self-acceptance. She is prepared to get on with her life, and is in a position to make a real choice about whether that life will include her spouse or not. The decision to stay is made not out of desperation or a fear of being left alone, but rather because she has forgiven her partner, values the relationship, and prefers to be in it than out of it. She no longer feels like a victim; in fact, she often feels that the difficulties she has endured as a result of her spouse's behavior have resulted in some inner changes that have been beneficial to her, whether she is still married or has ended the relationship.

Most offenders' spouses go through the above stages. However, therapy with the couple will vary depending on the couple's stage in life and the couple's relationship, spirituality, and life's goals.

REBUILDING THE COUPLE RELATIONSHIP

An intimate relationship can be only as healthy as the two people in it. Before the two are counseled together, each needs individual treatment. The wife or significant other needs to feel safe to say what she is really feeling and not be forced into considering the exploitative partner's needs first.

Both members of the couple have come to the relationship with unresolved family-of-origin issues. These issues, which may have initially attracted these two people to each other, have undoubtedly affected the marriage adversely in various ways. In the case of the exploitative professional, his childhood wounds have found expression in unethical behavior, which has led to a personal and professional crisis. This crisis provides an opportunity for both members of the couple to heal individually. If they choose to stay together, their relationship may ultimately benefit. Living through the consequences of professional sexual exploitation constitutes a difficult way of acquiring psychological health and an improved relationship, and no one would willingly choose this path. But having been forced into it, the couple that fully engages in the process can reap great rewards.

It is important for the treatment team to remember that the offender's family members are secondary victims who need attention as part of the treatment process. In addition to treatment or therapy, participation of the spouse or significant other in a twelve-step support group can be beneficial. So can involvement of the couple in a support group for couples.

Recovering Couples Anonymous (RCA) (P.O. Box 10172, St. Louis, MO 63105) is a twelve-step fellowship of couples who are recovering from the effects of any addiction, often more than one addiction. About half the couples have had addictive sexual disorders. In couples meetings, subjects are discussed that are of particular interest to couples and that are less likely to be discussed at A.A. or related meetings, such as rebuilding trust, how much to reveal to the partner about past behaviors and present struggles, healthy sexuality, and negotiating money issues. These meetings model for newly recovering couples how other couples are dealing with these issues. They are highly recommended for couples wishing to improve their relationship.

14

A Path to Wholeness

You hear my words. Hear too that there are other words than mine. These are not meant for hearing with the physical ear. Because you see only me, you think there is no Way apart from me. You are here to learn, not to collect historical information.

Indires Shah 1983, p. 47

We need to acknowledge that the seeds of violence are in every man; therefore their education should be devoted to training that out, not beating it in: that aggression is contagious, and that watching it, reading about it, and expressing it will never reduce it, and consequently all arguments for letting off steam are spurious and corrupt: that the passion if violence will always, must always, be someone weaker, smaller and lower in the hierarchy of violence, if not of suffering. As long as aggression is admired, so long will men be the victims of their own dreams and delusions and the danger around them.

Rosalind Miles 1991, p. 245

TAKING INVENTORY

The archetypal themes in Section II present human qualities that helping professionals carry in their work:

- The naive prince reminds professionals that naïveté is not innocence and professional education is never complete. In the effort to empathize and identify with those served, the professional may become ensnared in an attraction and interaction that was not contemplated or planned. Professional sexual misconduct may occur without intention or premeditation.

- The wounded warrior exhorts professionals to identify our own wounds, for they are a powerful reservoir of our unresolved vulnerability as well as our healing potential. They are the legacy we bring into our work as helping professionals, and are the source of our pain as well as our compassion; the reservoir of our hubris as well as our inspiration and creative expression.

- The self-serving martyr within the professional may turn a lament of self-pity and suffering servitude into a narcissistic pursuit of gratification in betrayal of our professional covenant to those we serve. The power of justified and rationalized departures from an ethical foundation should not be underestimated.

- The false lover is the addict within, the propensity to pursue sensory objects with self-will and significant consequence in pursuit of pleasure. Each of us has a part of ourselves that does not wish to age or to accept adult responsibility for our actions.

- The dark king is the chilling shadow aspect of the power professionals are granted as servants of the people.

- The madman cries out to remind us to be grateful for our health and ability to exercise discrimination in our own lives without the challenge of fighting a major mental disorder.

NATURAL HISTORY OF REHABILITATION
FROM PROFESSIONAL SEXUAL IMPROPRIETY

For over twenty thousand years, the father remained removed from
the interior of the family by ignorance of the role he played in
procreation, by exogamy, by his emotional need to differentiate
himself from the mother, and by being increasingly valued primarily for what he could hunt or otherwise produce from outside
himself. What erupted as the patriarchy was an *enantiodromia*—a
flipping into the opposite—with splitting from the feminine as the
chief characteristic. The patriarchy was not necessarily a reaction
against matriarchy; it was more likely the consequence of naturally
emerging factors inherent in the evolution of males and gave rise
to images of the archetypal father in the culture of the West
(Pedersen 1991).

At work, too, the professional metaphorically assumes the father role in relation to his patient or client. Both in the home and
in the work system, assumption of the father role, with its powers
and responsibilities, provides opportunities for unresolved wounds
to be played out as sexual exploitation. When this happens, the
exploitative professional has the opportunity to address the wound
and heal. There are at present no published studies that portray
the natural course of professional sexual misconduct and sexual
offense. Nor are there any controlled studies that compare treatment approaches for professional sexual offense. Based on more
than ten years of experience with more than three hundred patients presenting with these problems, we offer the following
collective description of the course we have seen these individuals
take.

CONFRONTATION STAGE

The initial period is one of denial, minimization, and rationalization. The professional uses his defenses to limit the potential
damage to his reputation, family, and professional practice. Complainants are commonly pathologized, blurred boundaries are ra-

tionalized, and investigation interviews are conducted with limited disclosure and compliance. If the professional is required to complete a mental health evaluation, he tries to limit the scope of inquiry, and offers as little collateral information as possible. Spouses, office staff, and professional friends are directly or indirectly encouraged to offer little information to the evaluator or investigation team.

If the professional is seeing a therapist, the therapist is encouraged to advocate for the professional by indicating that no major psychopathology is present and the complaints are a result of misunderstanding or situational stress.

If the professional is suffering from a sexual disorder or impulse control disorder, efforts are made to curtail his sexual behavior, especially in the professional arena.

CRISIS STAGE

The professional reaches the point where he can no longer deny that a problem exists and that he has engaged in a boundary violation. Acting out sexually may or may not be admitted at this juncture. Emotional numbness and efforts to control the damage predominate. This stage may also include anger, defiance, distorted thinking, and, finally, discovery of personal vulnerability.

GRIEF STAGE

The professional begins to come to terms with the ethical violation and professional sexual misconduct and/or professional sexual offense. Anger at those who reported the boundary violation and who precipitated intervention transforms into pain and deep personal sadness. The grief is very self-centered at first, and focuses on income, professional status, and family stature lost. As the consequences of professional sexual impropriety become manifest, the grief extends to mourning of losses. Dysthymia, depression, self-destructive behavior, substance abuse, or addiction may all intensify at this stage.

PERSONAL REHABILITATION STAGE

The professional begins to address issues in his personal life, and to work at improving his physical and mental health. Self-diagnosis and acceptance of impairment are initial treatment objectives, as are relief from acute pain and crisis. There is limited improvement in quality of life. Financial consequences and time away from family may precipitate family conflict and discord. Making fundamental decisions in a period of major life transition is discouraged.

PROFESSIONAL REHABILITATION STAGE

The professional begins to consider how he can realistically return to productive employment. He furthers his understanding of the dynamics of exploitation of power and position, and begins to develop victim empathy. Career counseling may lead to career transition or a change to nonprofessional pursuits. He is encouraged to work at achieving a balance between work and personal life.

GROWTH STAGE

The professional begins to explore new ways of living in his world. He has defined a new relationship with family, begun to have empathy and compassion for himself and others. He has begun to develop trust that he can and will maintain healthier personal boundaries, and relationships with others. Spirituality emerges. Improvement occurs in the quality of relationships with family, friends, and community. He now has greater comfort with employment, workplace, and other employees.

AUTHENTICITY STAGE

The professional begins to define his true self, and develops the courage and will to live in harmony with this image. Spiritual development is a focus at this stage. He feels a new freedom and is now able to uphold healthy boundaries for self and others. Healthy sexuality becomes a reality for him.

PROCEEDING WITH HEALING

How do we proceed with the healing? Our lives are replete with
self-guides, tapes, workbooks, websites, and other tools that might
help us find our way. Yet the path is as ephemeral as the concept;
the way is uncertain.

We cannot lead anyone further than we have gone ourselves.
We cannot teach what we have not learned, offer as wisdom what
we have not integrated and assimilated. We can speak of wholeness only to the extent that we have achieved it in our own lives.
But if we don't attempt to inspire and encourage the patient, we
remain spectators.

What would a path of wholeness for a helping professional
look like? How would it feel? Can one know when one's feet are
on the path or off? For a helping professional who has engaged
in professional sexual misconduct, is there genuine personal healing? Is restitution to victims and their families possible? Can family members, friends, peers, or the public forgive the professional
for ethical violation?

THE USE OF A CARTOGRAPHY

A cartography provides us with a multidimensional map of para-
digms and mental landscapes that are difficult to negotiate. One
of the more helpful things that can be undertaken is to develop
an understanding of the life pattern seen in human growth and
development. It is then possible to place oneself, or the person one
is treating or assisting, at an appropriate developmental point on
that spectrum. However, the task is rather daunting without guidance and the ability to understand and embrace one developmental
model to the point that it resonates with personal life experience.
Defining "normal" growth and development is as culturally, ethni-
cally, and religiously sensitive as defining "normal" eating patterns,
"healthy" sexuality, or "democratic" government. Yet without using
any guideline, in this case a multidimensional grid or cartography,
we would be consigned to finding our way alone without the benefit of the experience, strength, and hope others can provide.

Choosing a cartography is the important step. Translation of a model to the patient/helping professional/counselee is needed. Common psychoanalytic models include those by Mahler, Kernberg, and Kohut. Other models are those developed by Piaget, Maslow, Erikson, and Winnicott. We offer the reader our personal preference, that of Ken Wilbur.

Wilbur's model contains lines of human development (affective, cognitive, moral, ego, object relations, etc.), and several dozen levels or stages of development, through which each of the various lines may progress. Structures or formations of the psyche are divided into two general types: basic structures and transition structures (Wilbur et al. 1986). Basic structures are defined as those that, once they emerge in development, remain in existence as "units" in the course of subsequent development. Transition structures, in contrast, are developmental phase-specific, temporary structures that tend to be replaced during subsequent phases of development. Negotiating these structural developments is the self, which is the locus of personal identification, volition, will, defense, and navigation through the developmental system, that which experiences each level of struggle, growth, and development.

Now comes the key to the use of this or any other model: if the self is to ascend or evolve through a hierarchy of basic structural development—that is, to grow and mature—then eventually it must release or negate its exclusive identification with its present level in order to identify with the next higher level in the developmental ladder. According to Wilbur and colleagues (1986), the self must accept the "death," negation, or release of the lower level through detachment or disidentification with an exclusive involvement with that level. The lower stage is released and negated, but the basic structure remains in place as a necessary rung in the ladder of evolving consciousness.

The self must die or surrender old ways of being again and again through life. When this is not possible due to separation, isolation, fear, or trauma, then we are stuck at a particular level until we can accomplish certain important phase-specific tasks. Then through consolidation and integration, we have the opportunity to move on to where we will be challenged anew by other developmental tasks.

In the area of professional sexual misconduct, the work usually begins through the clinical investigation of problems with false or untenable belief systems regarding self and self-worth, cognitive distortions (particularly in object relations), and the recognition and protection of self and interpersonal boundaries. The more daunting and longer-term work invariably comes down to dynamic investigation of dysfunction with borderline and narcissistic disorders. These disorders are in contrast to the classical psychoneuroses (such as anxiety, hysteria, and obsession-compulsion), and require a different analytic approach. The major difference is that in the psychoneuroses there is some conflict or repression within the self structure (the ego would repress the id), whereas in borderline or narcissistic conditions there is too little self to perform such repression. In this situation, there is too little true Self, as it is obscured by the inflated ego of the narcissist or the fragmented ego of the borderline. Then the conflicts emerge as disruptive behavior, violence, exploitation of power, or other unskillful actions that paradoxically are self-defeating or self-destructive.

Such borderline and narcissistic conditions can be viewed as (1) character pathology that could become manifest at any developmental level, or (2) a pathological arrest or fixation to the expected narcissistic or borderline characterological features of some lower developmental structure (level) (Wilbur et al. 1986). The importance of this differentiation is that anyone can develop as a defensive pathology a morbid, overexpanded, or fragmented self structure at any given level of human development. Thus, many people with characterological pathology need not be seen as having a characterological curse that is immutable and fixed, particularly if they are using these features to work through a given developmental level.

The importance of the arguments expounded above is that without completing characterological growth and development there is limited potential for healing at more than a superficial level. Of course, the first goal for victim or perpetrator suffering from professional sexual exploitation is to stop the continuation of trauma and violence. Cognitive-behavioral treatment is essential for this goal. However, without the additional goal of growing as described in the preceding paragraphs, no personal evolution or transformation occurs. One remains bound to the trauma and violence even if it is no longer acted out behaviorally. The trauma and suffering fail to have meaning in life, and victim pathology and concretized characterological defenses are eventually manifested.

A practical way to approach this dynamic work is through exploration of personal cycles of ego expansion and deflation. For the purposes of this discussion, we will adopt the definitions of ego and Self used by Edinger (1972), wherein the Self is the ordering and unifying center of the total psyche, just as the ego is the center of the conscious personality. In other words, ego is the seat of subjective identity while the Self is the seat of objective identity.

GROWTH AND DEVELOPMENT
IN THE FIRST HALF OF LIFE

The task of the first half of life involves ego development with progressive separation between ego and Self, whereas the second half of life requires a surrender or at least an ability to put the ego in proper perspective as it experiences and relates to the Self.

In the first half of life, the developmental process is experienced as an alternation between two states of being—inflation and alienation. The term *inflation* describes the attitude and the state that accompany the identification of the ego with the Self. It is the state in which something small (the ego) has arrogated to itself the qualities of something larger (the Self) and hence is blown up beyond the limits of its proper size. The ego totally identified as the Self experiences itself as a deity.

A common example of ego inflation is a person whose grandiosity and idealism lead him to believe he is unique and has achieved a royal or divine status. Ego inflation can entail spells of anger; the urge to vengeance; power motivation of all kinds; intellectual rigidity, which attempts to equate its own private truth with

the universal truth; lust and all operations of the pure pleasure
principle; and any desire that considers its own fulfillment the central value. There is also negative inflation, which is associated with
identification with the divine victim—an excessive unbounded sense
of guilt and suffering, martyrdom and sacrifice for others.

The Matter with Mother

When the world is seen in black and white, a man often finds
himself wrestling with the archetypal forces of the mother complex.
When images of "good" or "bad" can be experienced as extensions
of Mother Earth and are accompanied by highly charged feelings
in relation to one's actual mother, a woman in authority, or a man's
wife, we say that he has a mother complex (Pedersen 1991). The
mother complex may be considered the most difficult encounter
a man ever faces. It is the regressive capacity in him and it will
destroy his life more quickly than any other single element in his
psychology. It is his wish to regress into infancy and be completely
indulged and taken care of by (m)others. When a man continues
his adolescent bravado and braggadocio into his adulthood, the
mother complex is unresolved. Dark moods, high-risk adventures,
and self-destructive actions are common symptoms as well.

The first developmental task is to understand that the mother
complex is not one's actual mother. It is also not uncommon for
a man to project his mother complex on an institution or profession where one can evade the responsibilities and struggles of adult
life (Johnson 1994).

Much of man's challenge in the middle of life is gained
through mindfully and consciously choosing to make the transition
from struggling against the regressive pull of the mother complex
(and at times giving into it) and coming to appreciate the spiritual and higher qualities of mother and the women who have been
in his life since. In them and through them a man may come to a
greater understanding of the feminine spiritual qualities of God and
of the archetypal mother. In other words, in midlife a man may
come to realize that his mother did the best she could, his lovers
in life are not copies of his mother, and that it is necessary to love

someone for who she is and not who she might resemble in some way. In the process, a man may develop genuine spirituality that identifies aspects of God that have qualities he considers feminine.

"A young man must make the transition from complex to archetype before he is capable of doing a man's work, occupying a place in the adult world, or forming any mature relationship" (Johnson 1994, p. 34).

Hubris

The Greeks had a tremendous fear of what they called *hubris*. The original usage of the term meant wanton violence or passion arising from pride. Hubris is the human arrogance that appropriates to man what belongs to the gods. It is the transcending of natural human limits. In this regard, it is a manifestation of ego inflation or expansion. Although the ego begins in a state of inflation, due to identification with the self, this condition cannot persist. Encounters with reality frustrate inflated expectations and bring about an estrangement between ego and self. This estrangement is symbolized by such images as a fall, an exile, a wound that cannot be healed, an ongoing source of despair or suffering. Not only has the ego been chastened, it has been injured.

Campbell (1949) eloquently described these masculine developmental cycles archetypally as a heroic journey, wherein the essential function of the heroic struggle and conflict is to develop an individual's proper "ego-consciousness," with progressively greater awareness of personal strengths and weaknesses. The hero's symbolic death becomes a marker of achievement of maturity.

Pedersen (1991) believes we can consider the classic hero's journey a form of initiation that attempts to provide access to a higher level of awareness by challenging the initiate with some task that involves eventually sacrificing different levels of ego dominance. Myths in which a fatherless young man sets out on a journey to find something of great value, to recapture something that was lost, or to find a new land, to solve a riddle that leads to some form of revelation or to bring about some cure or healing of himself are archetypal patterns of masculine development. These patterns act as metaphorical models of certain life experiences that need to be lived and integrated by individual men to facilitate the development of their consciousness and, eventually, a greater spiritual relation to life. This occurs through that part of the individuation process known as the transcendent function, a merging of the conscious and unconscious elements in such a way that there is a further constellation of the higher self.

According to Edinger (1972), psychic growth involves a series of inflated or heroic acts. These provoke rejection and are followed by alienation, repentance, restitution, and renewed inflation. This cyclic process repeats itself again and again in the early phases of psychological development, each cycle producing an increment in consciousness. The cycle can go wrong. It is subject to disturbances, especially in the early phases of life. The cycle can be blocked if sufficient acceptance and renewal of love did not occur. This creates a buildup of frustration and despair. Blockage can also occur if the environment of the child is so totally permissive that he has no significant rejection experiences at all, if the parents never say no. Then the whole experience of alienation is omitted and the child gets acceptance for his inflation. This leads to spoiled child psychology and contributes to a provisional life in which limitations and rejections have scarcely been experienced at all.

In the state of alienation, the ego is not only disidentified from the self, which is desirable, but also disconnected from it, which is most undesirable. When the connection is broken the result is emptiness, despair, meaninglessness, and in extreme cases psychosis or suicide. Whenever one experiences an unbearable alienation and despair, it is followed by violence. The violence can take an external or an internal form. In extreme cases this means either murder or suicide. The crucial point is that at the root of violence of any form lies the experience of alienation—a rejection too severe to be endured.

Jung (1953a) says essentially the same thing:

> The self, in its efforts at self-realization, reaches out beyond the ego-personality on all sides; because of its all encompassing nature it is brighter and darker than the ego, and accordingly con-

fronts it with problems which it would like to avoid. Either one's
moral courage fails, or one's insight, or both, until in the end
fate decides. You have become the victim of a decision made
over your head or in defiance of the heart. From this we can
see the numinous power of the self, which can hardly be expressed in any other way. For this reason the experience of the
self is always a defeat for the ego. [par. 778]

A classic symbol for alienation is the image of the wilderness. And
it is here, characteristically, that some glimpse of a spiritual awakening can be encountered.

THE SECOND HALF OF LIFE

Among all my patients in the second half of life (that is to say,
over 35) there has not been one whose problem in that last
resort was not that of finding a religious outlook on life. It is
safe to say that every one of them fell ill because he had lost
what the living religions of every age have given to their fol-
lowers, and none of them has been really healed who did not
regain his religious outlook. This course has nothing whatever
to do with a particular creed or membership of a church. [Jung
1953a, par. 509]

Edinger (1972) states that just as the experience of active inflation is a necessary accompaniment of ego development, so the
experience of alienation is a necessary prelude to awareness of the
self. This experience of being in the wilderness may be described
as a kind of neurosis, within which an individual questions his right
to exist, has a profound sense of unworthiness, and may believe
his innermost desires, needs, and interests must be wrong or unacceptable. His psychic energy is dammed up and may emerge in
covert, unconscious, or destructive ways, such as psychosomatic
symptoms, anxiety, depression, alcohol or substance dependency,
compulsive gambling, or an addictive sexual disorder. Fundamentally, such a patient is facing the problem of whether or not he is
truly a child of a divine power. To break out of the alienated state
some contact between ego and self must be reestablished.

The ego-inflated state, when acted out, leads to a fall and hence to alienation. The alienated condition, likewise under normal circumstances, leads to the state of healing and restitution. Inflation or alienation become dangerous conditions only if they are separated from the life cycle of which they are part. If either becomes a static, chronic state of being, the integrity of self and relation to other including the perception of a living divine power is threatened.

The central aim of all spiritually based religious practices is to keep the individual (ego) related to the deity. All religions are repositories of transpersonal experience and archetypal images. All religious practices hold up to view the transpersonal categories of existence and attempt to relate them to the individual. Religion is the best collective protection available against both inflation and alienation. So far as we know, every society has had such spiritual qualities in its collective life rituals. It is doubtful if humanity and civilization (as we know it) can survive for any period without some common, shared sense of awareness of these spiritual qualities. Like Edinger, we also believe that at a certain point in psychological development, usually after an intense alienation experience, the ego-self complex sustains a shift in perception or consciousness. The ego becomes aware, experientially, of a spiritual energy or force (which may be God) to which the ego is subordinate.

This is the central theme: Psychological development in all its phases is a redemptive process. The goal is to redeem by conscious realization, the hidden self, hidden in unconscious identification with the ego. The repetitive cycle of inflation and alienation is superseded by the conscious process of individuation when awareness of the reality of the ego-self complex occurs. Once the reality of the spiritual center has been experienced, a dialectic process between ego and self can, to some extent, replace the previous pendulum swing between inflation and alienation. But the dialogue of individuation is not possible as long as the ego thinks that everything in the psyche is of its own making. (Edinger 1972). This is the healing of the narcissistic and/or borderline characterological features of some developmental stage that precedes the integration, personal evolution, and transformation that occurs in a major personal developmental advance. But the fear of egoic death is difficult to overcome without support and encouragement, therapy, and commitment to a spiritual life and religious practice.

The same principles are expounded in the twelve-step addiction model of healing (Alcoholics Anonymous 1976). These seem to be much more accessible and practical for many individuals we have treated who have been either victims or perpetrators of professional sexual exploitation. Unconscious or preconscious unintegrated experiences, which we have called wounds, often take the form of compulsive or addictive behavior. These include the abuses and other traumas we suffer and then paradoxically reenact in a recurring repetition compulsion. We often hurt those whom we love, and defile that which we most value personally and professionally. In spite of these tragic consequences, the addictive behavior may represent the only way such experiences may reach consciousness, be resolved, and allow one to find deeper meaning in life. In the twelve-step programs these concepts are referred to as "hitting bottom," "cleaning house," and "having a spiritual awakening."

It is in mindfully experiencing the tension between living the provisional life in its superficial and mundane daily course, and touching the archetypal patterns that stir our souls as they emerge from the unconscious, that we feel a sense of authenticity of self and direction in our lives. This direction is symbolized by major emotional experiences and life passages, which we consider turning points. Maslow (1968) referred to those events that positively change our lives as peak experiences. Even if an experience feels more like descending into a valley or abyss, rather than climbing a mountain top, who can really say that it may not serve to aid us in our life journey and personal growth. These events usually have some archetypal core, which is related to our parents or some other key developmental issue. Jung referred to this ongoing process as the path of individuation (Pedersen 1991).

Paradoxically, at the very time when a person comes to realize how little he knows about unconditional love, selfless service,

authenticity, equanimity, and genuine spirituality, there is the opportunity to find deeper meaning and truer, clearer perceptions.
This can and must be addressed by the sexually exploitative professional or those in his family or vocational system. Will, reason,
and imagination are distinctively human faculties that allow sex to
actualize itself as anatomic contact and in some instances as eros
in human beings. Animals have sex; human beings have the capacity for reflection on this biological phenomenon as a part of a
relationship with another (human) object.

Allan Bloom (1993) writes:

> One cannot ignore man's imaginative and rational contribution
> to his own formation. . . . Coupling begins as sexual desire but
> often has as its end (ideal) love. The various kinds of love af-
> fairs, like the various kinds of political orders, are human be-
> ings' often inept attempts to realize inchoate potentialities that
> are specific to man. Without examining the ends these associa-
> tions aimed at, no one can give an adequate account of them.
> [pp. 19–20]

This requires those who would adjudicate, punish, or diagnose
the sexually exploitative professional to remember always that in
the unmasking of the pain and suffering that the result of sexual
desire acted out can have upon our lives and souls, we strive to do
more than simplify and civilize the raging, confusing, and chaotic
feelings associated with such acts. It is far from easy to differentiate
between the delicate interplay of giving one's body or private interests and thoughts to someone else in order to gain respect, trust,
and assistance. If this should occur within a fiduciary relationship
between a professional and one served, the complexity can be seen
when the art of helping as a professional becomes mixed with the
arts of eros and seduction, the toxins of anger and lust. The Greeks
believed that eros is a natural longing for the beautiful that can
be corrupted and misplaced, but remains itself a noble passion.

It is the position of Jungian psychology that behind the great
myths of the world and all of life's important and oft-repeated
experiences are their archetypes in the collective unconsciousness.
A particular archetype may rule or dominate a great deal of the

ego's life. For each great peak-and-valley experience of life, each great transition or occasion, each passage, there is an archetype. An innate capacity for self-delusion and self-destruction is built into the human psyche. Although the concept of free will was debated in Greek philosophy, virtually all agreed that the will was not free to choose without a knowledge of good, and that ignorance was almost certain to lead to evil. Walter Otto (1981) argues that it is virtually impossible to distinguish between the will of a human being and the power of a deity in Greek thought; what a man wills and does is himself and is the deity. Both are true, and in the last analysis the same.

If a power over which we have no control enters our minds and hearts, and urges us toward a sinful or ruinous course of action, then in what sense can we be held responsible for what we did? One answer has to do with what the Greeks called the "spiritual eye." Through this eye, people can become aware of the influence of a god upon them. They can also discern the consequences of their actions. But for the eye to be effective, they must also have seen the three great Greek realities: the nature of the beautiful, the just, and the reasonable. If people can develop and hold what we would call a capacity for conscious insight, for true values, and for "right order," then they need not be so possessed that they are driven to acts of sin or destruction. For the Greeks the concept of an operative conscience on one hand and the idea of spiritual and psychological awareness on the other belong together.

The qualities that would cloud over the spiritual eye were Ate and hubris. According to Sanford (1995), Ate instills in human hearts a wanton disregard both for morals and for the consequences of our actions. It is she who confuses our minds and so blinds us spiritually that we not only act with a disregard for what is morally right but also for our own long-term self-interest. Bewildered by reckless impulse, we are led to our ruin. As the story goes, Ate was thrown out of Olympus after she had tricked and deceived Zeus. Since then she has wandered over the world, inciting human beings to acts of folly, ruin, and sin by destroying their good judgment, confusing their minds, and obliterating their moral sensibilities. The earth itself was called by the ancients the meadow of Ate. It was said that she never walked on the ground, but on the heads of mortals. In many stores dealing with Ate, we find that a fatal inclination toward Ate was able to possess a person because that person had succumbed to the sin of hubris, an exaggerated arrogance provoked by excessive pride. To the Greeks, it denoted a wanton violence and insolence resulting in disdainful arrogance, which causes a person to despise the laws of the state and the moral imperatives.

Putting this into psychological language, we would say that the fantasy leading up to an action and the impulse toward an action that would follow from the fantasy come from an archetype. Such an action might be good and creative, but it might be evil and destructive. If the ego is stirred up or infected by an archetype, then that archetype will possess or dominate the person and impel him or her toward a certain typical course of action. To the extent that the ego is blind to the profound unconscious spiritual influences at work in his or her psyche, then there is effectively little or no free will, but if a person has at least a modicum of psychological insight and spiritual awareness and some warm connections to other human beings, then the capacity to choose one's actions is still possible.

The developmental task at hand is to mature and grow an observing ego, which can not only exist and react in the midst of life events, and respond to fantasy or urge, but also have the capacity to observe itself and make necessary corrections in action and thought. The development of these powers of self-observation greatly strengthens the ego against otherwise blind compulsions thrust upon it from certain archetypes, and the fantasies and effects that they engender. Both a relevant spiritual life and effective psychotherapy will support development of an observing ego.

Our defense would seem to depend on three things:

- our state of moral and psychological awareness
- some sense of moral and spiritual values
- the quality of our relationships with other human beings.

This same concept was discussed in analytical rather than mythological terms by Jung (1953b) in his letter to Bill Wilson: "I am strongly convinced that the evil principle prevailing in this world leads the unrecognized spiritual need [in the alcoholic] into perdition, if it is not counteracted by either a real religious insight or by the protective wall of human community. An ordinary man, not protected by an action from above and isolated in society, cannot resist the power of evil [addiction]" (p. 624).

FINDING THE FAIR WITNESS

The difficult task each of us faces is to identify and then effectively utilize an observing ego that can serve as our daimon, an attendant spirit or "genius within," our inner gyroscope that will help us stay on course in our life. It is in some respects an identification with the inner wisdom of the soul. This function is also referred to by some Buddhists as the development of the fair witness, or "the still small voice within" described in the Old Testament. With the evolution of a mature ego that is neither inflated nor fragmented, it is possible to put our own problems and successes, liabilities and gifts in proportion to those of the remainder of humanity. We find ourselves as we find our place in the human community. It is at this point that we can begin to appreciate the inner and deeper meanings of many of our human dramas.

It is now possible to explore the inner meaning of the metaphor of incest as it relates to professional sexual misconduct. In this regard incest is the psychological act of turning the flow of instinctual energy back upon itself. As the Self, the part of one that strives toward ideals and goals, is able to see the self in unskillful action and thought, mindfulness and freedom from violence is won. Caution must be used. This search for redemption must be undertaken with the care and support of others who are experienced in the inner journey.

> Incest, molestation, and sexual exploitation are graphic examples of the golden touch of an emerging inner consciousness being acted out unconsciously in pathological and destruc-

tive ways. It is absolutely essential that our capacity for "incest"
be used [and explored] on its creative [personal, symbolic]
level—that of creating consciousness and culture. It should be
safeguarded from its literal expression, which is so destructive
to the human psyche. Any who misunderstand or cheat, refus-
ing to pay the cost of inner growth, pay instead in the coin of
loneliness, anxiety, and alienation.

One of the noblest acts a man can perform is to keep his consciousness at a level and direction appropriate to his current
stage of development. To pretend he is more advanced than
he really is causes psychological splits; yet to refuse to grow
always forces someone else to pay his psychological debts. And
eventually he also will pay for what has been acted out consciously or unconsciously. [Johnson 1991, pp. 28, 45]

An Indian story that parallels the oedipal myth reveals a quite
different attitude toward femininity. A small segment of the
Mahabharata, the story of Nala and Damayanti, offers us another
perspective on the balance between masculine and feminine values. In it the strength of the feminine, the woman as hero, is the
redeeming factor. We cannot be charged for fate, for it is not of
our making, but the manner in which we proceed with that fate is
our responsibility. Damayanti avoids the romantic fantasy of a god
as a lover. This requires a finely tuned ability to make psychological and emotional distinctions. At a particular point in her life she
chooses the limited human over the divine. Femininity may serve
masculinity, but this must be understood as an interior dynamic
and not as an external, relational convention. When she uses her
masculine quality of differentiation, she does so in the service of
her genius for relatedness. It is her capacity to act when required
and to endure when that is appropriate that produces the redemptive power (Johnson 1991).

In human life the individual achieves significance through discrimination and the setting of limits. Therefore what concerns
us here is the problem of clearly defining these discriminations,
which are, so to speak, the backbone of morality. Unlimited

possibilities are not suited to man; if they existed, his life would only dissolve in the boundless. To become strong, a man's life needs the limitations ordained by duty and voluntarily accepted. The individual attains significance as a free spirit only by surrounding himself with these limitations and by determining for himself what his duty is. [I Ching Hexagram 60]

CONCLUSION: MEETING THE CHALLENGE OF AN OCCUPATIONAL HAZARD

In the life of every professional are times of trial and temptation. Although it may at first seem inconceivable, the majority of helping professionals have at some point in their career faced a situation in which a choice needed to be made between an action that would be in their personal interest and fulfill their desire or fantasy, and an alternative that was in the best interest of the person they were serving.

Peter Rutter (1989), in his book *Sex in the Forbidden Zone*, suggests that in the very act of exploiting a woman in order to feel more alive, the man in power "abandons his search for aliveness within himself" (p. 22). For many women under the influence of such a "forbidden zone" relationship, there was a definite nonsexual value placed on the relationship before any sexual activity took place. Confusion then developed between sexual activity as an act and as a symbol for intimacy and the achievement of a complete relationship. Rutter states that for the man in power, the underlying psychological reality that leads to exploitation is that he is as likely to be ministering to his own wounds as those of the woman he uses. The quest for healing frequently takes such men to women for sexual contact. There men experience their injuries with depression, hatred, inadequacy, meaninglessness, and the losses associated with their behavior. When these psychological wounds are denied (submerged) the anima may be projected outward with qualities of receptivity, vulnerability, and a desire to nurture and be nurtured. Then sexual fantasy and the thrill of the unknown and forbidden may lead to obsessions, destructive and self-defeating behavior, and sexual contact.

Rutter (1989) describes such a moment from his own psychiatric practice with courage and candor in his book introduction:

> Nothing in my training had prepared me for this moment. As
> Mia moved closer to me, I sat frozen, neither encouraging her
> nor stopping her. I was overcome by an intoxicating mixture
> of the timeless freedom, and the timeless danger, that men feel
> when a forbidden woman's sexuality becomes available to them.
> The freedom stems from the illusion of such moments in which
> a man can convince himself that nothing but sexual merger
> with the female body and spirit seems real. He shuts himself
> off from past and future, contemplating neither his motivation
> nor the consequences of his acts. The feeling of danger bal-
> ances the one of freedom, for within this danger is the intu-
> ition that the act he is so strongly fantasizing may be wrong,
> that it may bring catastrophe on both himself and the woman.
> In the moment of deciding whether to cross the line, I felt all
> at once extremely powerful—and very, very vulnerable. [p. 4]

He goes on to say that when a man in power relinquishes his
sexual agenda toward a woman under his care in order to preserve
her right to a nonsexual relationship, a healing moment occurs for
both parties. For some women, the healing moment was explicit—
discussed, acknowledged, and relinquished. For others, the fact that
the man in power never related to her sexually when she was vulnerable to seduction provided the healing without any verbal ac-
knowledgment or expression. The man in power then simultaneously or subsequently creates a moment for himself in which he
realizes that the release of this woman from his secret desire that
she heal him, also liberates him from the endless suffering associated with pursuit of sexual gratification.

This inherent occupational hazard lies at the base of every professional admonition that stretches back into the origins of the
helping professions: a professional in power remains human and
thus fallible to an error in judgment in which the desire to be
himself comforted and gratified overshadows the professional ethics required to safely and effectively be of service to another.

Contemplation of this truth regarding professional service requires each helping professional and those served to look upon the professional–patient relationship more carefully. Is it realistic to expect and even demand that each professional be flawless in the performance of his duties? Is a professional responsible not only for the results of his actions but also for being human, harboring within certain inherent imperfections? How can a professional maintain the inspiration and courage to serve if any error in judgment could end his career?

The trauma of professional sexual misconduct and sexual offense is serious and violates not only ethics but also the ability to trust within fiduciary relationships. Yet without the ability to risk within such relationships, their power for healing, personal transformation, and benefit is seriously depleted. Protection and preservation of the ability for both the professional and the person served to risk must be fostered. To react to the current controversy regarding male abuse of power with rigid protectionism and boundaries that do not allow for individual expression and response to a person's request for help and understanding would be almost as devastating as having poorly defined professional ethical expectations and standards. The public needs protection, but at some point the price of increased protection is interference with the ineffable qualities of such fiduciary relationships and the features that make them meaningful and effective.

We are brought to the point in this contemplation where one must consider what can be done. Perhaps through the archetypal themes presented, and the powerful lessons we can learn from those who exploit power and position through sexual behavior and those who suffer from such violations, we can be more thoughtful in our own roles in life as professionals and as those served by others. We can have compassion and recognize the variety of personal problems and mental disorders, the wounds that may have been present in each before such behavior was acted out, and how the manifestation of violation and exploitation added to these wounds.

And perhaps we can come to recognize that only through education of professionals and consumers can we change the prevalence of this violence. The provision of an ongoing dialogue in which abuse of power and sexual violence can be discussed is needed in professional training programs, continuing professional education, public forums, and regulatory agencies.

We cannot legislate or enforce an end to exploitation and violence. We can bring it out of the darkness. We can continue to provide the opportunity for individuals to risk and to trust in their relationships with professionals.

References

Ackerman, D. (1994). *A Natural History of Love*. New York: Random House.

Alcoholics Anonymous. (1976). *Alcoholics Anonymous*, 3rd ed. New York: Alcoholics Anonymous World Services.

American Bar Association. (1998). *Model Rules of Professional Conduct*. Chicago, IL: American Bar Association.

American Psychiatric Association. (1989). *The Principles of Medical Ethics with Annotations Especially Applicable to Psychiatry*. Washington, DC: American Psychiatric Association.

———— (1994). *Diagnostic and Statistical Manual of Mental Disorders, Fourth Edition*. Washington, DC: American Psychiatric Association.

Applebaum P., Jorgenson, L., and Sutherland, P. (1994). Sexual relationships between physicians and patients. *Archives of Internal Medicine* 154:2561–2565.

Barth, R. J., and Kinder, B. N. (1987). The mislabeling of sexual impulsivity. *Journal of Sex and Marital Therapy* 13:15–23.

Bennett, B. E., VandenBos, G. R., and Greenwood, A. (1990). *Pro-*

fessional Liability and Risk Management. Washington, DC: American Psychological Association.

Blanchard, G. T. (1991). Sexually abusive clergymen: a conceptual framework for intervention and recovery. *Pastoral Psychology* 39:237–246.

Bloom, A. (1993). *Love and Friendship.* New York: Simon & Schuster.

Bly, R. (1989). Male naiveté and the loss of the kingdom. *Pilgrimage* 15(5):2–14.

——— (1990). *Iron John: A Book About Men.* Woburn, MA: Addison-Wesley.

Bowlby, J. (1973). *Separation: Anxiety and Anger.* New York: Basic Books.

Brien, D., ed. (1995). *Mirrors of Transformation: The Self in Relationship.* Berwyn, PA: Round Table.

Briere, J. (1992). *Child Abuse Trauma: Theory and Treatment of the Lasting Effects.* Newbury Park, CA: Sage.

Campbell, J. (1949). *The Hero with a Thousand Faces.* Princeton, NJ: Princeton University Press, Bollingen Series.

Carnes, P. (1983). *Out of the Shadows: Understanding Sexual Addiction.* Center City, MN: Hazelden.

——— (1991). *Don't Call It Love.* New York: Bantam.

Coleman, E. (1990). The obsessive-compulsive model for describing compulsive sexual behavior. *American Journal of Preventive Psychiatry and Neurology* 2:9–14.

Corey, G., Corey, M. S., and Callanan, P. (1993). *Issues and Ethics in the Helping Professions.* Pacific Grove, CA: Brooks/Cole.

Council on Ethical and Judicial Affairs, American Medical Association (1991). Sexual misconduct in the practice of medicine. *Journal of the American Medical Association* 266:2741–2745.

Diagnostic and Statistical Manual of Mental Disorders (1994). 4th ed. Washington, DC: American Psychiatric Association.

Edinger, E. (1972). *Ego and Archetype.* Boston, MA: Shambhala.

Engel, H. G. (1987). Physicians' sexual feelings toward patients. *Medical Aspects of Human Sexuality*, pp. 41–48.

Epstein, R. S., and Simon, R. I. (1990). The exploitation index: an early warning indicator of boundary violations in psychotherapy. *Bulletin of the Menninger Clinic* 54:450–465.

Erikson, E. (1950). *Childhood and Society.* New York: Norton.

Ethics Committee, American Psychiatric Association. (1986). Psychiatrist–patient sexual contact. *American Journal of Psychiatry* 143:1149.

Fortune, M. (1989a). Betrayal of the pastoral relationship. In *Psychotherapists' Sexual Involvement with Clients: Intervention and Prevention,* ed. G. Schoener, J. Milgrom, J. Gonsiorek, et al., pp. 84–93. Minneapolis, MN: Walk-in Counseling Center.

——— (1989b). *Is Nothing Sacred?* San Francisco, CA: HarperCollins.

——— (1995). Is nothing sacred? When sex invades the pastoral relationship. In *Breach of Trust,* ed. J. C. Gonsiorek, pp. 29–40. Thousand Oaks, CA: Sage.

Fossum, M. A., and Mason, M. J. (1986). *Facing Shame: Families in Recovery.* New York: Norton.

Gabbard, G. (1995). Psychotherapists who transgress boundaries with patients. In *Breach of Trust: Sexual Exploitation by Health Care Professionals and Clergy,* ed. J. Gonsiorek, pp. 136–144. Thousand Oaks, CA: Sage.

Gabbard, G., and Lester, E. (1995). *Boundaries and Boundary Violations in Psychoanalysis.* New York: Basic Books.

Gabbard, G., and Nadelson, C. (1995). Professional boundaries in the physician–patient relationship. *Journal of the American Medical Association* 273(18):1445–1449.

Gartrell, N., Herman, J, Olarte S., et al. (1986). Psychiatrist–patient sexual contact: results of a national survey, I. Prevalence. *American Journal of Psychiatry* 143:1126–1131.

Gartrell, N. K., Milliken N., Goodson, W. H., et al. (1992). Physician–patient sexual contact: prevalence and problems. *Western Journal of Medicine* 157:139–143.

Gonsiorek, J. (1995). Assessment for rehabilitation of exploitative health care professionals and clergy. In *Breach of Trust: Sexual*

Exploitation by Health Care Professionals and Clergy, pp. 145–162. Thousand Oaks, CA: Sage.

Greenson, R. (1968). Dis-identifying from mother: its special importance for the boy. *International Journal of Psycho-Analysis* 49:370–378.

Gutheil, T. (1991). Patients involved in sexual misconduct with therapists: Is a victim profile possible? *Psychiatric Annals* 21:661–667.

Gutheil, T. G., and Gabbard, G. O. (1993). The concept of boundaries in clinical practice: theoretical and risk management dimensions. *American Journal of Psychiatry* 150:188–196.

Guyon, R. (1934). *The Ethics of Sexual Acts*. New York: Knopf.

Henderson, J. (1964). Ancient myth and modern man. In *Man and His Symbols*, ed. C. Jung, p. 128. New York: Doubleday.

Hudson, L., and Jacot, B. (1991). *The Way Men Think: Intellect, Intimacy, and the Erotic Imagination*. New Haven, CT: Yale University Press.

Hunter, M., and Struve, J. (1997). *The Ethical Use of Touch in Psychotherapy*. Thousand Oaks, CA: Sage.

Irons, R. (1991). Contractual provisions for professional re-entry. *American Journal of Preventive Psychiatry & Neurology* 3(1):57–59.

Johnson, R. (1991). *Femininity Lost and Regained*. New York: Harper Perennial.

——— (1994). *Lying with the Heavenly Woman: Understanding and Integrating the Feminine Archetypes in Men's Lives*. New York: HarperCollins.

Jorgenson, L. M. (1995). Sexual contact in fiduciary relationships: legal perspectives. In *Breach of Trust*, ed. J. C. Gonsiorek, pp. 237–283. Thousand Oaks, CA: Sage.

Jung, C. G. (1953a). Mysterium conjunctionis. In *Collected Works* 1953, vol. 14, par. 778

——— (1953b). *C. G. Jung's Letters*, vol. 2. Princeton, NJ: Princeton University Press.

Kerenyi, K. (1974). *The Gods of the Greeks*, trans. N. Cameron. London: Thames and Hudson.

Kernberg, O. (1986). Factors in the treatment of narcissistic personalities. In *Essential Papers on Narcissism*, ed. A. P. Morrison, pp. 236–239. New York: New York University Press.

Legg, A., and Legg, D. (1995). The offender's family. In *Restoring the Soul of the Church*, ed. N. M. Hopkins, and M. Laaser. Minneapolis, MN: Liturgical Press.

Levine, S., and Levine, O. (1995). *Embracing the Beloved.* New York: Doubleday.

Love, P. (1990). *The Emotional Incest Syndrome.* New York: Bantam.

Lowen, A. (1967). *The Betrayal of the Body.* New York: Macmillan.

Mahler, M. S., Pine, F., and Bergman, A. (1975). *The Psychological Birth of the Human Infant.* New York: Basic Books.

Miles, R. (1991). *Love, Sex, Death, and the Making of the Male.* New York: Simon & Schuster Summit Books.

Moore, T. (1992). *The Care of the Soul.* New York: HarperCollins.

Moore, R., and Gillette, D. (1992a). *The King Within.* New York: William Morrow.

———— (1992b). *The Warrior Within.* New York: William Morrow.

Morrison, A. (1986). Shame, ideal self and narcissism. In *Essential Papers on Narcissism*, pp. 365–372. New York: New York University Press.

Morrison, J. (1995). *The DSM-IV Made Easy.* New York: Guilford.

New York State Bar Association Code of Professional Responsibility (1992). Albany, NY: New York State Bar Association.

Nouwen, H. (1992). *The Return of the Prodigal Son: A Story of Homecoming.* New York: Doubleday.

Otto, W. (1981). *Dionysus: Myth and Cult.* Dallas, TX: Spring.

Oxford Book of English Verse (1940). Oxford: Oxford University Press.

Patai, R., and Patai, J. (1989). *The Myth of the Jewish Race*, 2nd ed. Detroit, MI: Wayne State University Press.

Pedersen, L. (1991). *Dark Hearts: The Unconscious Forces That Shape Men's Lives.* London: Shambhala.

Pope, K. S. (1988). How clients are harmed by sexual contact with mental health professionals: the syndrome and its prevalence. *Journal of Counseling and Development* 67:222–267.

Pope, K. S., Keith-Spiegel, P., and Tabachnick, B. (1986). Sexual attraction to clients: the human psychologist and the (sometimes) inhuman training system. *American Psychologist* 41:147–158.

Pope, K. S., Levenson, H., and Schover, L. R. (1979). Sexual intimacy in psychology training: results and implications of a national survey. *American Psychologist* 34:682–689.

Ravagli, A., and Weekly, C. M., eds. (1964). *The Complete Poems of D. H. Lawrence.* New York: Viking.

Ross, L. B., and Roy, M., eds. (1995). *Cast the First Stone: Ethics in Analytic Practice.* Wilmette, IL: Chiron.

Rutter, P. (1989). *Sex in the Forbidden Zone.* Los Angeles: Jeremy Tarcher.

———— (1996). *Sex, Power, & Boundaries.* New York: Bantam.

Sanford, J. A. (1995). *Fate, Love, and Ecstasy: Wisdom from the Lesser Known Goddesses of the Greeks.* Wilmette, IL: Chiron.

Schneider, J., and Irons, R. (1996). Differential diagnosis of addictive sexual disorders using the *DSM-IV. Sexual Addiction & Compulsivity* 3:7–21.

Schneider, J., and Schneider, B. (1990). *Sex, Lies, and Forgiveness: Couples Speaking on Healing from Sex Addiction.* Center City, MN: Hazelden Educational Materials.

Schoener, G. R. (1995). Assessment of professionals who have engaged in boundary violations. *Psychiatric Annals* 25(2):95–99.

Schwartz, M. F. (1995). In my opinion: victim to victimizer. *Sexual Addiction & Compulsivity* 2:81–88.

Shah, I. (1983). *The Way of the Sufi.* New York: Norton.

Simon, R. I. (1997). Boundaries in psychotherapy: a safe place to heal. *Harvard Mental Health Letter* June, pp. 4–5.

Sontag, S. (1989). *AIDS and Its Metaphors.* New York: Farrar, Straus, & Giroux.

———— (1995). *Illness as Metaphor.* New York: Doubleday.

State Bar of California—Rules of Professional Conduct (1995). Sacramento, CA: State Bar of California.

Stoller, R. (1974). Symbiosis, anxiety, and the development of masculinity. *Archives of General Psychiatry* 30:164–169.

Storr, A. (1996). *Feet of Clay: Saints, Sinners, and Madmen: A Study of Gurus.* New York: Simon & Schuster.

Torrey, E. F. (1986). *Witchdoctors and Psychiatrists.* New York: Harper & Row.

Unitarian-Universalist Association. (1993). (Jan/Feb.): *The World*, p. 25.

Unitarian-Universalist Ministers' Association. (1997). Code of Professional Practice. Boston, MA: U. U. Ministers' Association.

University of Arizona. (1997). *Code of Academic Integrity*, revised. Tucson, AZ: University of Arizona.

Von Franz, M. (1981). *Puer Aeternus.* Boston, MA: Sigo.

Washton, A. (1989). Cocaine may triger sexual compulsivity. *US Journal of Drug and Alcohol Dependency* 13:8.

Welwood, J. (1996). *Love and Awakening: Discovering the Sacred Path of Intimate Relationship.* New York: HarperCollins.

Wilbur, K., Engler, J., and Brown, D. (1986). *Transformations of Consciousness: Conventional and Contemplative Perspectives on Development.* Boston: New Science Library.

Zweig, C., and Abrams, J., eds. (1991). *Meeting the Shadow: Hidden Power of the Dark Side of Human Nature.* New York: Tarcher/Putnam.

Credits

The authors gratefully acknowledge permission to reprint material from the following sources:

Diagnostic and Statistical Manual of Mental Disorders, Fourth Edition. Copyright © 1994 American Psychiatric Association.

"Sexual Misconduct in the Practice of Medicine," *Journal of the American Medical Association*, vol. 266, pp. 2741–2745. Copyright © 1991 by the American Medical Association.

"The Offender's Family," by A. Legg and D. Legg, in *Restoring the Soul of the Church*, edited by N. M. Hopkins and M. Laaser. Copyright © 1995 by Liturgical Press.

Dark Hearts: The Unconscious Forces That Shape Men's Lives, by L. Pedersen. Copyright © 1991 Shambhala Publications.

A Natural History of Love, by Diane Ackerman. Copyright © 1994 Random House.

Index

Abrams, J., 26, 137, 165, 168, 169
Ackerman, D., 28, 48, 54, 176
Addictions
  desire and, 95
  self-serving martyr, 145–147
  sexual addiction and, 45–46
  sexual disorders and, 31–46. *See also* Sexual disorders
  treatment for, xii–xiii
Aichhorn, A., 66
Alcoholics Anonymous, 44, 45, 86, 120, 162, 209, 225
American Association of Pastoral Counselors, 5
American Bar Association, 79, 80
American Medical Association, 5, 68, 72, 75
American Psychiatric Association, 5, 54, 68, 73

American Psychological Association, 68
Anger, family of offender, 200–205
Applebaum, P., 72
Attorney–client relationship, professional sexual misconduct, 79–81
Attraction to clients, sexually exploitative relationship, 55–56
Authenticity stage, rehabilitation, 215

Bennett, B. E., 56
Bipolar affective disorder, *DSM-IV*, 40–41
Blame, family of offender, 194–197
Blanchard, G. T., 51
Bloom, A., 226
Bly, R., 103, 109